Safe Orthopaedic Surgery

S. Venkatesh Babu

Safe Orthopaedic Surgery

The Anatomic Principles and Techniques for Preventing Complications

Springer

S. Venkatesh Babu
Consultant Orthopaedic and Trauma surgeon
Sri Sakthi Hospital
Tirunelveli, India

Expert Committee Member in Trauma Surgery
The Tamilnadu Dr MGR Medical University
Tamilnadu, India
e-mail: drsvbabu@hotmail.com

ISBN 978-981-16-2848-1 ISBN 978-981-16-2846-7 (eBook)
https://doi.org/10.1007/978-981-16-2846-7

This Springer imprint is published by the registered company Springer Nature Singapore Pte Ltd.
The registered company address is: 152 Beach Road, #21-01/04 Gateway East, Singapore 189721, Singapore

Foreword

The phrase "primum non nocere" or "first do no harm "has been part of medical culture for thousands of years. First appearing in some versions of the Hippocratic Oath the phrase became popularized by Auguste Chomel in the eighteenth century. The last hundred years has seen a rapid expansion in the treatment of many conditions especially the advent of operative surgery in the treatment of fractures and the principle of safety in surgery—doing no harm—has become more and more important.

This book focusses on the complications that can occur during and after surgery and most importantly what the surgeon and the operating team can do before during and after the surgical procedure.

The book is divided into twelve anatomical regions with an additional chapter on the safe use of antibiotics—a topic of vital importance in the developing world. Each chapter describes the applied surgical anatomy of the region under discussion and outlines the key surgical approaches use to treat lesions in that area. The text stresses the close relationship between anatomy and surgical approaches and shows how to avoid complications.

Many chapters describe in detail the complications that can occur and the text is complemented by a series of anatomical diagrams that illustrate key anatomical features relevant to the surgery that needs to be performed.

The book is an important perspective in the concept of safe surgery.

Mr Piet deBoer MA FRCS
Former Director of Education, AO Foundation, Davos, Switzerland
Author, Many Books including Surgical Exposures in Orthopaedics
Walters Kluwer & LWW
Visiting Lecturer, University of Rijeka Medical School, Republic of Croatia
Honorary Consultant Orthopaedic Surgeon, York Hospital, United Kingdom

Preface

Since my medical school years and residency days, I have observed the confidence of surgeons who have both the vast anatomic knowledge and precise skills required to produce excellent results and happy patients. Miller's pyramid is a method of ranking clinical competence in educational settings and the workplace. The pyramid is broken into four levels: *knows, knows how, shows how,* and *does*. To gain the surgical technique and skills to be competent, a surgeon must go through a learning curve from knows to does. A surgeon has to become an expert in the field to be a safe doctor!

This was of such interest to me that I wrote my thesis on the theme of safe surgery for my MCh Orth degree course in the United Kingdom. Although the region where I practice has limited resources, I strive to keep my orthopaedic knowledge and skills up to date by reading relevant journals and periodically attending orthopaedic forums. I noticed that the meetings and publications always include a session or article on complications. Having accumulated notes on safety facts for all my surgeries over the past 20 years, I was invited to deliver a lecture on complications of clavicle fracture surgery at a regional orthopaedics meeting. My talk on the finer details of preventing surgical complications was well appreciated, and that night I thought of publishing my notes on safely performing all the orthopaedic fracture surgeries for the benefit of both surgeons and patients. Hence, this book was born!

The report "To Err Is Human" was published by the Institute of Medicine in 1999 and drew the attention of both surgeons and the public. Despite the many benefits of orthopaedic surgery for managing pathologies, the discipline is associated with many potential complications. It has been calculated that the cumulative probability of having a wrong-site surgery at least once in an orthopaedic surgeon's lifetime career is 25%. Studies have shown that surgeons and gynecologists have a lower life expectancy than clinicians, and emotional stress is one reason for this difference. Surgical complications are a real cause of stress in surgeons. Thus, we need to take the utmost care in preventing technical hitches considering that both patients' and our own lives are involved.

It is my sincere belief and hope that *Safe Orthopaedic Surgery* will support all orthopaedic surgeons and create safer surgery for all orthopaedic patients.

Tirunelveli, India

S. Venkatesh Babu, MCh Orth., MBA, FRCS
e-mail: drsvbabu@hotmail.com

Contents

About the Author

S. Venkatesh Babu is an internationally trained orthopaedic and trauma surgeon from India. He is an active member of state, national, and international orthopaedic and trauma surgical bodies. Dr. Babu has given many presentations at international forums and had multiple publications in orthopaedic journals. He was also instrumental in organizing Golden Hour Trauma Care through the Highway Emergency Clinics, providing ambulance service to regions of India with fewer resources. Dr. Babu is currently the Chief Orthopaedic & Trauma Surgeon at Sri Sakthi Hospital in Tirunelveli City, India. He is an Expert Committee Member in Trauma Surgery at the Tamilnadu Dr MGR Medical University.

Safe Use of Antibiotics in Orthopaedic Surgery

1

1.1 Introduction

The World Health Organization (WHO) estimates that more than 50% of antibiotics in many countries are used inappropriately. In its latest advisory, WHO suggested the adoption of "access, watch, and reserve," an approach that specifies which antibiotics to use for the most common and serious infections (access), which to have available at all times in the healthcare system (watch), and which to use sparingly or reserve for last resort (reserve). WHO has urged all countries to adopt these guidelines to reduce antimicrobial resistance, adverse events, and treatment costs [1].

Orthopaedic surgery is a unique and growing speciality that requires the utmost care to prevent infection. The efficacy of prophylactic antibiotics has been well established in orthopaedic surgery [2]. They are effective at reducing infection when administrated just before the surgical incision is made. The multiple studies referenced in the NICE Guidelines, and the standards of the British Association of Plastic, Reconstructive and Aesthetic surgeons have confirmed this efficacy in joint arthroplasty, fracture surgery, and spine surgery [3–5]. Nevertheless, surgical site infections continue to be a major source of morbidity, mortality, and hospital costs [6, 7].

The combination of incorrect use of antibiotics and easy access fuels antibiotic resistance, which is a growing concern both in India and worldwide. A recent study confirmed the overuse of antibiotics in India, with a high antibiotic prescription rate in the private sector [8]. This study also highlighted that primary care physicians in the private sector can play a key role in reducing antibiotic misuse and overuse [8].

Through the Indian Council of Medical Research and National Centre of Disease Control, the Health Department of the government of India has provided guidelines for antimicrobial use that focus on effectiveness and cost reduction. These guidelines advise the precise choice of antibiotics and duration of use in all specialities, including infectious diseases and orthopaedic and fracture surgery [9, 10].

S. V. Babu, *Safe Orthopaedic Surgery*,
https://doi.org/10.1007/978-981-16-2846-7_1

1.2 Microorganism Prevalence and Antibiotic Therapy in Orthopaedic Surgery

According to the 2017 guidelines from the Indian Medical Council Research and other studies, *Staphylococcus aureus*, coagulase-negative staphylococci, and gram-negative bacilli are the predominant microorganisms associated with acute osteomyelitis, septic arthritis, and surgical site infections after spine surgery, arthroplasty, fracture surgery with internal fixation devices, functional tissue repair, and trauma [9–17]. In external fixation, the most common organisms causing infection are *S. aureus*, *Staphylococcus epidermidis*, and *Escherichia coli*, especially in children.

The overall incidence of orthopaedic surgical site infection ranges from 0.8 to 71% [15]. Surgical site infection in implant surgery has an incidence of 2–22% and is a serious complication, leading to increased morbidity and higher treatment costs [15]. The increasing incidence of road traffic accidents and traumatic injuries in India is contributing more open fractures that require antibiotics [16].

Table 1.1 covers specific organisms and the proper choice of antibiotics in orthopaedic and trauma surgery.

Table 1.1 Microorganisms and choice of antibiotics in orthopaedic and trauma surgery

Disease/ challenge	Microorganisms	First choice	Second choice	Duration
Cellulitis, soft tissue infection, lymphangitis	Group A streptococci, *Streptococcus pyogenes*, *Staphylococcus aureus*	Cloxacillin 50–100 mg/kg/d in 3–4 divided doses, *or* Co-amoxiclav 1.2 g BD, *or* Cefazolin injection 50 mg/kg/d in BD	Clindamycin 600 mg q 8 h in penicillin-allergic patients	5–7 days
Acute osteomyelitis, septic arthritis	Group A streptococci, *S. pyogenes*, *S. aureus*	Co-amoxiclav 1.2 g BD, *and* Gentamycin 80 mg	Ceftriaxone injection 1 g, *with or without* Vancomycin injection 1 g	4–6 weeks
Chronic osteomyelitis	Multiple organisms, including gram-negative bacilli, anaerobes	Pathogen-specific antibiotics after culture and bone biopsy	–	>6 weeks
Surgical site infection, implant surgery infection	*S. aureus* and coagulase-negative staphylococci and gram-negative bacilli	Ceftriaxone 2 g IV OD *with* Vancomycin injection 1 g IV BD	Teicoplanin injection 800 mg 3 doses over 12 h followed by 400 mg once daily	4 weeks
Open fracture	*S. aureus* and coagulase-negative staphylococci and gram-negative bacilli	Co-amoxiclav 1.2 g BD, *or* Cefuroxime 1.5 g q 8 h	Clindamycin 600 mg q 8 h in penicillin-allergic patients	Until wound debridement

1.3 Antibiotic Prophylaxis in Orthopaedic and Trauma Surgery

Prophylactic antibiotic administration is valuable for reducing infection and sepsis after orthopaedic surgery. Antibiotics are usually administered intravenously 15–30 min before surgery begins. However, some evidence suggests that antibiotics are not needed for orthopaedic surgery that does not involve soft tissue or implants [2]. For open fractures, antibiotic prophylaxis and antitetanus measures are typically provided in the emergency department. The recommended antibiotics are continued until wound debridement (excision; Table 1.2) [2–4, 9, 18, 19].

1.4 Antibiotic Stewardship Programs in Orthopaedic Surgery

Antibiotic stewardship programs (ASPs) are currently recommended in all medical establishments to manage surgical site infections through judicious use of antibiotics [20]. The goals of these program are to decrease hospital-acquired infections, control costs, and prevent complications associated with antibiotic usage (e.g., renal damage, *Clostridium difficile* infections). ASPs use a multidisciplinary team consisting of surgeons, infectious disease specialists, clinical pharmacists, and infection control and prevention practitioners [6]. The efficacy of such programs has been shown, with good results in challenging microorganisms and reducing infections [4, 5, 6, 20], leading to improved patient outcomes and cost-effective medical care [5, 20, 21].

ASPs provide expert guidance on judicious usage of antibiotics, including the following:

- Determining appropriate indications of antibiotic administration
- Choosing the correct antibiotic based on known or expected pathogens
- Determining the correct dosage
- Determining the appropriate duration of treatment

Table 1.2 Prophylactic antibiotics in orthopaedic and trauma surgery

Orthopaedic and closed fracture surgery	Cefuroxime injection 1.5 g IV STAT and BD for 24 h (maximum) *or* Cefazolin injection 2 g IV STAT and BD for 24 h
Trauma and open fracture surgery	Cefuroxime injection 1.5 g IV STAT and BD for 24 h (maximum) *or* Cefazolin injection 2 g IV STAT and BD for 24 h The antibiotics are continued until wound debridement (excision)

1.5 Discussion

Both patient and procedural factors can contribute to surgical infections. Patient factors include age, immunosuppression, diabetes mellitus, anemia, smoking, prolonged hospital stay, coexisting infections at other sites, obesity, malnourishment, and carriage of resistant organisms. Procedural factors include surgical technique, longer duration of surgery, inadequate hemostasis, variations in body temperature, skin antisepsis, operating room ventilation and air changes, presence of foreign body, tissue trauma, and preoperative shaving of hair [15, 18].

A high index of suspicion for infection should be maintained for 3 months following orthopaedic surgery. The choice of antibiotics for surgical site infections depends on the antibiotic susceptibility of the causative organism. The antibiotic chosen must cover the main contaminant flora present in the skin or mucosa disrupted by the incision. The most effective, least toxic, and least expensive antibiotic administered for a precise duration of time is what should be used to prevent or cure infection.

Bacterial eradication should be the primary goal of antibiotic therapy. Microbiologic diagnosis is vital because using antibiotics for nonbacterial infections risks development of bacterial antibiotic resistance, and correct diagnosis of specific bacterial infection is the key to limiting unnecessary prescribing.

Clinicians must prescribe antibiotics empirically but intelligently. Pharmacokinetics and pharmacodynamics come into play when choosing the most effective agent and dosage. Consider local resistance, efficacy, and cost-effectiveness. Encourage patient compliance. For patients with recurrent infections, consider taking microbiologic samples and reviewing the antimicrobial prescription when the results are available. Avoid treatment for colonization without evidence of infection unless there is a clear indication in the guidelines.

References

1. World Health Organization (2017, June 6) WHO updates essential medicines list with new advice on use of antibiotics, and adds medicines for hepatitis C, HIV, tuberculosis and cancer. https://www.who.int/news/item/06-06-2017-who-updates-essential-medicines-list-with-new-advice-on-use-of-antibiotics-and-adds-medicines-for-hepatitis-c-hiv-tuberculosis-and-cancer
2. Oishi CS, Carrion WV, Hoaglund FT (1993) Use of parenteral prophylactic antibiotics in clean orthopaedic surgery: a review of literature. Clin Orthop Relat Res 296:249–255
3. Nanchalal J, Nayagam S, Khan U, et al (2009) Standards for the management of open fractures of the lower limb. British Association of Plastic, Reconstructive and Aesthetic Surgeons website. https://www.bapras.org.uk/docs/default-source/commissioning-and-policy/standards-for-lower-limb.pdf?sfvrsn=0
4. National Institute for Health and Care Excellence (2019) Surgical site infections: prevention and treatment. NICE guideline 125. https://www.nice.org.uk/guidance/ng125
5. National Institute for Health and Care Excellence (2015, August 18) Antimicrobial stewardship: systems and processes for effective antimicrobial medicine use. NICE guideline 15. https://www.nice.org.uk/guidance/ng15

6. Campbell KA, Stein S, Looze C, Bosco JA (2014) Antibiotic stewardship in orthopaedic surgery: principles and practice. J Am Acad Orthop Surg 22(12):772–781
7. Rajkumari N, Gupta AK, Mathur P et al (2014) Outcomes of surgical site infections in orthopaedic trauma surgeries in a tertiary care centre. J Postgrad Med. 60(2):254–259
8. Farooqui HH, Mehta A, Selvaraj S (2019) Outpatient antibiotic prescription rate and pattern in the private sector in India: evidence from medical audit data. PLoS One 14(11):e0224848
9. National Centre for Disease Control (2016) National treatment guidelines for antimicrobial use in infectious diseases. Directorate General of Health Services, Ministry of Health and Family Welfare, Government of India. https://ncdc.gov.in/WriteReadData/l892s/File622.pdf
10. Indian Council of Medical Research, Department of Health Research (2017) Treatment guidelines for antimicrobial use in common syndromes. https://iamrsn.icmr.org.in/images/pdf/STG270217.pdf
11. Leekha S, Terrell CL, Edson RS (2011) General principles of antibiotic therapy. Mayo Clin Proc 86(2):56–167
12. Salkind AR, Rao KC (2011) Antibiotic prophylaxis to prevent surgical site infections. Am Fam Physician 83(5):585–590
13. Chahoud J, Kanafani Z, Kanj SS (2014) Surgical site infections following spine surgery: eliminating the controversies in the diagnosis. Front Med (Lausanne) 1:7
14. Ceroni D, Grumetz C, Desvachez O et al (2016) From prevention of pin-tract infection to treatment of osteomyelitis during paediatric external fixation. J Child Orthop 10(6):605–612
15. Amaradeep G, Shiva Prakah SS, Manjappa CN (2017) Surgical site infections in orthopaedic implant surgery and its risk factors: a prospective study in teaching hospital. Int J Orthop Sci 3(3):169–172
16. Home (Transport) Department, Government of Tamil Nadu (2019, January) Road accident analysis in Tamil Nadu. https://tnsta.gov.in/pdf/analysis_jan2019.pdf
17. Rehmus WE (2021) Cellulitis. MSD manual consumer version. https://www.msdmanuals.com/home/skin-disorders/bacterial-skin-infections/cellulitis
18. Dryden M (2019) Surgical antibiotic prophylaxis. Surgery (Oxford). 37(1):19–25
19. Soriano A, García-Ramiro S, Mensa J (2007) Antimicrobial prophylaxis in orthopaedic surgery. In: Meani E, Romanò C, Crosby L et al (eds) Infection and local treatment in orthopedic surgery. Springer, Berlin, pp 49–57
20. World Health Organization (2019) Antimicrobial stewardship programmes in health-care facilities in low- and middle-income countries: a WHO practical toolkit. https://www.who.int/publications/i/item/9789241515481
21. Seligman KM, Katz D, Farber MK (2018) Preventing surgical site infection after cesarean delivery: the anesthesia professional's role. APSF Newsl 33(1):25–27

Safe Clavicle Fracture Surgery 2

2.1 Introduction

A fall on the outstretched arm or a direct blow to the shoulder representing an axial compressive force on the clavicle is the most common mechanism of clavicle fracture [1, 2]. Clavicle fractures account for 2.6–5% of all fractures in adults and 10–15% of fractures in children [3]. The most common site for this fracture (80%) is in the middle third of the clavicle, where it is displaced in 73% of patients [4]. The distal end fracture has a 21–28% incidence, with 10–52% being displaced [5], and the medial end constitutes only 2% of all clavicle fractures [6].

The goal of clavicle fracture treatment is to achieve healthy bony union without any dysfunction, cosmetic deformity, or other morbidity [7]. Management varies depending on location and displacement.

The approach to management of displaced middle-third clavicle fracture has changed in recent years. In a Canadian study, adult patients treated conservatively showed higher rates of nonunion than those treated surgically [8]. Moreover, patient-reported outcome measures that detect even subtle loss of function in daily activities have favored operative management [9–11]. The two most important meta-analyses of randomized clinical trial results concluded that surgical fixation yielded better outcomes than conservative treatment for displaced middle-third clavicle fractures, including in regard to fracture healing and appearance [7, 12]. Thus, nonsurgical management is reserved for midshaft clavicle fractures without displacement.

Placement of a titanium elastic nail has proved to be safe, less invasive, and trustworthy for displaced, noncomminuted midshaft clavicle fractures in adolescents [13]. Because of the unbalanced nature of the lateral-third clavicle fracture, surgical treatment is justified and has good functional outcome [5, 14–17]. Despite the rarity of medial-third clavicle fractures, there are a few noteworthy reports indicating that

S. V. Babu, *Safe Orthopaedic Surgery*,
https://doi.org/10.1007/978-981-16-2846-7_2

surgery is indicted, especially in children, for open fractures with broad soft tissue damage, when there is neurovascular injury, and for sternoclavicular dislocation [6, 11, 18–20].

2.2 Applied Surgical Anatomy of the Clavicular Region

Insufficient knowledge of anatomy and inability to recognize key structures can lead to grave complications in surgery [21]. Major complications of clavicle fracture surgery have been reported in recent decades [3, 4, 7, 22–27], including fatal complications such as vascular injuries and pneumothorax [18, 28]. Good knowledge of the applied anatomy of the operative region combined with expert skills has been shown to yield better results [6, 27, 29]. The following review of applied anatomy is provided as a refresher for the surgeon who is going to manage clavicle fractures in a safe manner (Fig. 2.1).

A distinctively twisted long bone, the clavicle measures 13.5–14.5 cm in length and 17 mm in thickness, with a S-shaped cephalad-to-caudad curvature. The middle shaft of the bone is relatively thin, unsupported by ligaments, and moderately unprotected, making it the most susceptible area to fracture. The clavicle is close to important vital structures, including the brachial plexus, which is 20 mm away, and the subclavian artery, which is 18 mm from the middle third. The subclavian vein lies immediately behind the medial clavicle. The pleura extends well up into the supraclavicular space in the process of inspiration.

The exact clavicle length should be maintained during fracture surgery for optimal results.

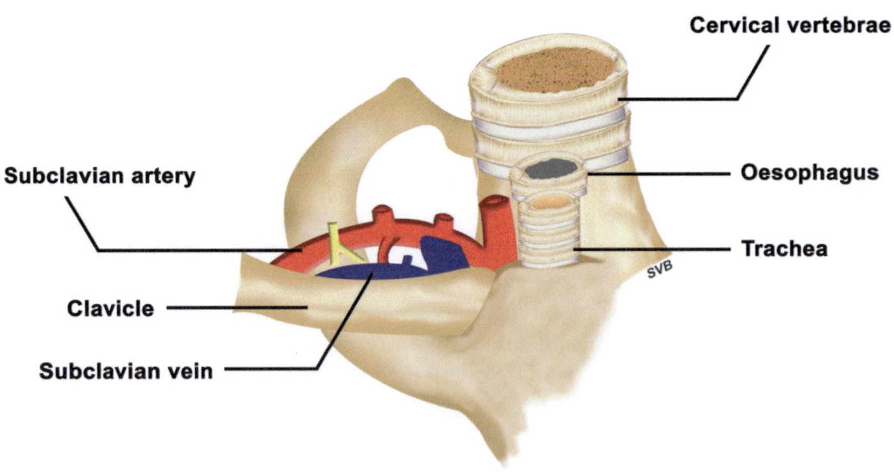

Fig. 2.1 The clavicle and its vascular relations

2.3 Principles of Safe Clavicle Fracture Surgery [4, 24, 28, 29]

2.3.1 Safety Principles for Preoperative Planning and Anaesthesiology

- The explanation of strategies to the anaesthesiologist in regard to the operation, alternate plans, and potential complications is of supreme importance. It will help them be prepared in case of emergency.

2.3.2 Safety Principles for Patient Positioning

- The beach chair position nicely provides anterior and lateral accessibility to the shoulder joint. An image intensifier is a great aid. However, the posterior approach to the shoulder is difficult in the beach chair position, and this position should not be used in medically compromised patients. The patient's head must be in neutral position, and close monitoring of the brain's perfusion pressure is indicated in longer surgeries to avoid neurologic injury, cardiac insult, or embolism occurrence.
- The supine position permits combined surgical approaches for a polytrauma patient but is limited to anterior shoulder surgeries only.
- Regardless of the patient position chosen, the table setup must allow the anaesthesiologist and operating team to rapidly alter the position in the event of emergency.

2.3.3 Safety Principles for the Surgical Incision

- The incision for clavicle surgery must respect the Langer's line. It should not be directly on the clavicle but rather just below the bone.

2.3.4 Safety Principles for the Surgical Approach

- The anterior approach is for anterior and superior clavicular plating with an oblique 8–10-cm incision.
- For nailing, a 1–2-cm incision is made just anterolateral to the sternoclavicular joint. Blunt dissection to bone is made to expose the entry point of the nail. A same-sized incision is also made just below the middle third fracture site in case of open reduction.
- For minimal invasive plate osteosynthesis (MIPO), an anterior approach is used for diaphyseal clavicle fractures requiring anterior and superior plating. Two separate skin incisions, each 2–3 cm in length, are made over the lateral and medial ends of the clavicle, corresponding in position to the ends of the prese-

lected plate. A subcutaneous tunnel is made using blunt dissection connecting the medial and lateral incisions. Stab incisions are made directly over the plate holes for insertion of screws; similar same stab incisions are made for the pins and pointed reduction forceps.
- A superior approach to the clavicle can be used for all lateral, medial, and diaphyseal clavicle fractures with an oblique 8–10-cm incision made superiorly over the clavicle centered over the fracture site.

2.3.5 Safety Principles for the Plane of Surgical Exposure

- The release of soft tissues must be very gentle and subperiosteal. There are special instruments available that will protect the vital structures during clavicle surgery.

2.3.6 Safety Principles for Drill, Screw Direction, and Depth

- Given that the thickness of the clavicle is 17 mm, the screw length in the plate osteosynthesis should not be longer than this.
- For fixing a medial-third clavicle fracture, the drill and screws must be placed in a superior-to-inferior direction.
- For fixing a middle-third clavicle fracture, the drill and screws must be placed in an anterior-to-posterior direction.

2.4 Specific Injuries in Clavicle Surgery and Their Management [4, 8, 18, 24, 25, 28, 30–34]

2.4.1 Subclavian Artery Injury

Incidence: Uncommon.
Presentation: Life-threatening bleeding palpable pulsatile swelling, upper limb ischemia.
Level: First part of subclavian artery near a medial- or middle-third clavicle fracture.
Management: Hypovolemia correction and addressing hemothorax or pneumothorax; CT angiography with repair of vessel; finally, fixation of fracture.

2.4.2 Brachial Plexus Injury: Traction, Compression, and Entrapment

Incidence: 1% of clavicle fractures.
Presentation: Paresthesia and/or pain with posterior and middle branch involvement.
Level: Middle-third clavicle fracture.

Management: MRI; recovery in a few months or neurolysis/nerve transfers if required.

2.4.3 Pneumothorax and Hemothorax

Incidence: 3% of clavicle fractures.
Presentation: Associated scapular fracture, upper rib fracture, reported in open reduction and internal fixation (ORIF), dyspnea and surgical emphysema.
Level: Middle-third clavicle fracture.
Management: Intercostal drainage; fixation of fracture at later time.

2.4.4 Subclavian Vein Injury

Incidence: Rare occurrence during primary surgery and usually due to callus compression or attempt to remove callus.
Presentation: Life-threatening as pulmonary embolism or venous thrombosis; decrease in SPO_2 and hypercapnia; negative intrathoracic pressure.
Level: Medial-third clavicle fracture.
Management: Submerging the wound in normal saline, occlusive dressing, vascular expertise, careful removal of callus causing compression.

2.4.5 Other Vessel Injuries

Pseudoaneurysm: Presents as limb-threatening ischemia; treated with vascular graft or stent; excellent outcome.
Arteriovenous fistula: Presents as congestive heart failure or limb ischemia.
Venous injury: Air embolism; decrease in end tidal CO_2, decrease in SPO_2; aggressive fluid loading.

2.4.6 Refracture

Incidence: 4% following the removal of clavicular plate.
Level: Middle-third clavicle fracture.
Management/prevention: Retain plate 12–18 months; avoid sports activity for 3 months after plate removal.
Risk factors: Alcoholism and communited fractures (and of course nonunion follows!).

2.4.7 Thoracic Outlet Syndrome

Incidence: Rare; can be vascular or neurogenic; occurs mostly after conservative management of clavicle fractures (malunion), seldom in ORIF cases.

Presentation: Altered sensation, venous congestion, discoloration of the limb, compression at the costoclavicular space.
Management: Excision of callus, resection of clavicle, corrective clavicle osteotomy surgery, first rib resection, anterior and middle scalenectomy without rib resection.

2.5 Discussion

The clavicle is an unique bone that is very closely related to neurovascular structures and the thorax. Injury to these vital structures during surgery can lead to significant morbidity and mortality. Although the AO principles of fracture management [30] recommend clavicle surgery primarily for significantly displaced (>20 mm) midshaft clavicle fractures, associated subclavian vessel injury, brachial plexus injury, ipsilateral scapular neck fracture, and painful nonunion of clavicle fracture, there are many extended indications [3, 4, 11, 22, 24, 35–37].

Clavicle fractures are currently fixed mainly with plate osteosynthesis, intramedullary fixation, and Kirschner wires. The complications and functional outcome are same for late fixation and intramedullary fixation, but the former is associated with more neurovascular complications [34]. Many surgeons have reported neurovascular complications with plate osteosynthesis, including the legendary Dr. Neer [3, 4, 7, 18, 22–28].

Reporting complications and adverse outcomes following orthopaedic surgery has a crucial role in patient safety and is receiving increasing attention. The overall complication rate after orthopaedic surgery is 12.7% in a well-established orthopaedic center, and following of standard protocol improves safety and standard of care [27]. Supervised residents in a teaching institution can perform surgery as safely as senior orthopaedic surgeons [27].

It is highly recommended that all health establishments implement an antibiotic stewardship program and safety protocols to prevent and manage surgical site infections [38–41] (see also Chap. 1).

References

1. Stanley D, Trowbridge EA, Norris SH (1998) The mechanism of clavicular fracture: a clinical and biomechanical analysis. J Bone Joint Surg (Br) 70B:461–464
2. Nowak J, Malimin H, Larsson S (2000) The etiology and epidemiology of clavicular fractures: a prospective study during a two-year study in Uppsala, Sweden. Injury 31:353–358
3. van der Meijden OA, Gaskill TR, Millett PJ (2012) Treatment of clavicle fractures: current concepts review. J Shoulder Elbow Surg 21(3):423–429
4. Hillen RJ, Burger BJ, Pöll RG et al (2010) Malunion after midshaft clavicle fractures in adults: the current view on clavicular malunion in the literature. Acta Orthop 81(3):273–279
5. Sambandam B, Gupta R, Kumar S, Maini L (2014) Fracture of distal end clavicle: a review. J Clin Orthop Trauma 5(2):65–73
6. Smelt J, Khakha RS, Harrison-Phipps K et al (2017) An isolated traumatic medial third clavicular fracture requiring surgical fixation. Ann Thorac Surg 103(3):e297–e298

7. Qin M, Zhao S, Guo W et al (2019) Open reduction and plate fixation compared with nonsurgical treatment for displaced midshaft clavicle fracture: a meta-analysis of randomized clinical trials. Medicine 98(20):e15638
8. Altamimi SA, McKee MD (2008) Nonoperative treatment compared with plate fixation of displaced midshaft clavicular fractures: surgical technique. J Bone Joint Surg Am 90(Suppl 2, Pt 1):1–8
9. McKee MD, Pedersen EM, Jones C et al (2006) Deficits following nonoperative treatment of displaced midshaft clavicular fractures. J Bone Joint Surg Am 88A(1):35–40
10. Pecci M, Kreher JB (2008) Clavicle fractures. Am Fam Physician 77(1):65–70
11. Charles ER, Kumar V, Blacknall J et al (2017) A validation of the Nottingham Clavicle Score: a clavicle, acromioclavicular joint and sternoclavicular joint-specific patient-reported outcome measure. J Shoulder Elbow Surg 26(10):1732–1739
12. McKee RC, Whelan DB, Schemitsch EH, McKee MD (2012) Operative versus nonoperative care of displaced midshaft clavicular fractures: a meta-analysis of randomized clinical trials. J Bone Joint Surg Am 94(8):675–684
13. Bithrey JW, van der Merwe JF (2017) Outcomes of treatment of displaced midshaft clavicle fractures in adolescents using titanium elastic nails. SA Orthop J 16(3):55–61
14. Sajid S, Fawdington R, Sinha M (2012) Locking plates for displaced fractures of the lateral end of clavicle: potential pitfalls. Int J Shoulder Surg 6(4):126–129
15. Elgazar AS (2015) Fixation of lateral clavicle fractures by simple K-wires. Al-Azhar Assiut Med J 13(3 Suppl 2):91–98
16. Kapil-Mani KC, Acharya P, Arun S (2018) Precontoured clavicular locking plate with broad lateral end: a newly designed plate for lateral third clavicle fractures. Malays Orthop J 12(1):15–20
17. Ejagwulu FS, Lawal YZ, Maitama IM et al (2019) Management of clavicle fractures and adjacent clavicular joint dislocations in a tertiary health center, North West, Nigeria. Niger J Basic Clin Sci 16(1):15–23
18. Skedros JG, Knight AN, Mears CS, Langston TD (2014) Temporary sternoclavicular plating for an unusual double clavicle fracture (medial nonunion, lateral acute) complicated by an intraoperative pneumothorax. Case Rep Orthop 206125:1–5
19. Barrera-Ochoa S, Nuñez JH, Domenech-Fernandez P et al (2018) Medial third clavicular fracture in combination with a posterior sternoclavicular dislocation in skeletally immature patients: 2 cases of a new proximal clavicular injury. JSES Open Access 2(1):97–99
20. Frias M, Ramos R, Bernardes M et al (2018) Medial clavicle fracture dislocation surgically treated: case report. Trauma Cases Rev 4:066
21. Megrina JF, Wasson MN (2018) Avoiding complications in endoscopic surgery. Contemporary Ob/Gyn website. https://www.contemporaryobgyn.net/view/modern-medicine-feature-avoiding-complications-endoscopic-surgery
22. Kitsis CK, Marino AJ, Krikler SJ, Birch R (2003) Late complications following clavicular fractures and their operative management. Injury 34(1):69–74
23. Liu PC, Hsieh CH, Chen JC et al (2008) Infection after surgical reconstruction of a clavicle fracture using a reconstruction plate: a report of seven cases. Kaohsiung J Med Sci 24(1):45–49
24. Mouzopoulus G, Morakis E, Stamatakos M, Tzurbakis M (2009) Complications associated with clavicular fracture. Orthop Nurs 28(5):217–224
25. Millett PJ, Hurst JM, Horan MJ, Hawkins RJ (2011) Complications of clavicle fractures treated with intramedullary fixation. J Shoulder Elbow Surg 20(1):86–91
26. Pal CP, Dinkar KS, Shakunt RK et al (2018) Comparison of the functional outcome of intramedullary nailing versus plating in displaced midclavicular fractures. J Orthop Allied Sci 6(1):13–16
27. Willhuber GC, Stagnaro J, Petracchi M et al (2018) Short-term complication rate following orthopedic surgery in a tertiary care center in Argentina. SICOT J. 4:26
28. Clitherow HDS, Bain GI (2015) Major neurovascular complications of clavicle fracture surgery. Shoulder Elbow 7(1):3–12
29. Theelen L, Bischoff C, Grimm B, Heyligers IC (2018) Current practice of orthopaedic surgical skills training raises performance of supervised residents in total knee arthroplasty to levels equal to those of orthopaedic surgeons. Perspect Med Educ 7:126–132

30. AO Surgery Reference (2019). https://www2.aofoundation.org/wps/portal/surgery
31. Smekal V, Deml C, Irenberger A et al (2008) Length determination in midshaft clavicle fractures: validation of measurement. J Orthop Trauma 22(7):458–462
32. Yoo MF, Seo JB, Kim JP, Lee JH (2009) Surgical treatment of thoracic outlet syndrome secondary to clavicular malunion. Clin Orthop Surg 1:54–57
33. Ishimaru D, Ogawa H, Sumi H, Shimizu K (2012) Late thoracic outlet syndrome after clavicle fractures in patients with multiple trauma: a pitfall of conservative treatment. Open Journal of Orthopedics 2(3):90–93
34. Beliaev AM, Fougere C (2015) Thoracic outlet syndrome secondary to a mid-clavicle malunion. BMJ Case Rep 2015:bcr2015209583
35. Hussain N, Sermer C, Prusick PJ et al (2016) Intramedullary nailing versus plate fixation for the treatment displaced midshaft clavicular fractures: a systematic review and meta-analysis. Sci Rep 6:34912
36. Gille J, Schulz AP, Wallstabe S et al (2010) Hook plate for medial clavicle fracture. Indian J Orthop 44(2):221–223
37. Ruedi TO, Murphy WM (eds) (2000) AO principles of fracture management. Thieme, New York
38. World Health Organization (2019) Antimicrobial stewardship programmes in health-care facilities in low- and middle-income countries: a WHO practical toolkit. https://www.who.int/publications/i/item/9789241515481
39. National Institute for Health and Care Excellence (2015, August 18) Antimicrobial stewardship: systems and processes for effective antimicrobial medicine use. NICE guideline 15. https://www.nice.org.uk/guidance/ng15
40. National Institute for Health and Care Excellence (2019) Surgical site infections: prevention and treatment. NICE guideline 125. https://www.nice.org.uk/guidance/ng125
41. Seligman KM, Katz D, Farber MK (2018) Preventing surgical site infection after cesarean delivery: the anesthesia professional's role. APSF Newsl 33(1):25–27

Safe Shoulder Surgery 3

3.1 Introduction

The glenohumeral joint is a versatile joint that relies on a complex network of bony ligamentous, musculotendinous, and neurovascular structures for proper function. Injuries arising from dysfunction are common and potentially devastating. While many of these injuries can be managed conservatively, when surgical treatment is indicated, a thorough understanding of the anatomy of the shoulder girdle and related structures is critical. It is also important for the surgeon to be aware of commonly used arthroscopic and surgical approaches and methods of avoiding injury [1].

Frequently performed shoulder surgeries include reconstruction for instability, acromioplasty, subacromial decompression, fracture fixation, and arthroplasty. While technically challenging, arthroscopic shoulder techniques have become more and more common over the past three decades. Although arthroscopy has numerous advantages over open surgery, the complication rate is higher than with open procedures [2]. Moreover, arthroscopy of the shoulder has a higher rate of vascular and neurologic complications than arthroscopy of the knee. The "learning curve" theory in orthopaedic surgery, and more specifically in arthroscopic procedures, has been well addressed. The surgical complication rate of arthroscopic procedures is between 7.9 and 9.5% [2]. Complications include stiffness/arthrofibrosis, persistent pain, infection, nerve palsy, and vascular injury. Even wrong-side surgery had been reported [3]. Studies show that extensive surgical experience is associated with a reduced rate of technical hitches [2, 3].

Total shoulder arthroplasty is associated with fewer complications than open reduction and internal fixation (ORIF) and thus can be an important option in complex proximal humeral fractures in geriatric patients [4].

S. V. Babu, *Safe Orthopaedic Surgery*,
https://doi.org/10.1007/978-981-16-2846-7_3

Neurologic complications are common during shoulder surgery. Nerve injuries occur in 1–2% of patients who are undergoing rotator cuff surgery, in 1–8% of patients undergoing surgery for anterior instability, and in 1–4% of patients undergoing arthroplasty [5]. Moreover, thorough knowledge of nerve anatomy is indispensable during arthroscopy for secure portal placement and safe guidance of trocars to avoid nerve injury.

3.2 Applied Surgical Anatomy of the Shoulder

During shoulder surgery, the axillary nerve is most susceptible to injury because of its proximity to the inferior shoulder capsule (Fig. 3.1). Surgical insult by direct laceration is quite possible [3], so knowledge of and attention to joint anatomy are crucial to safe and successful surgery.

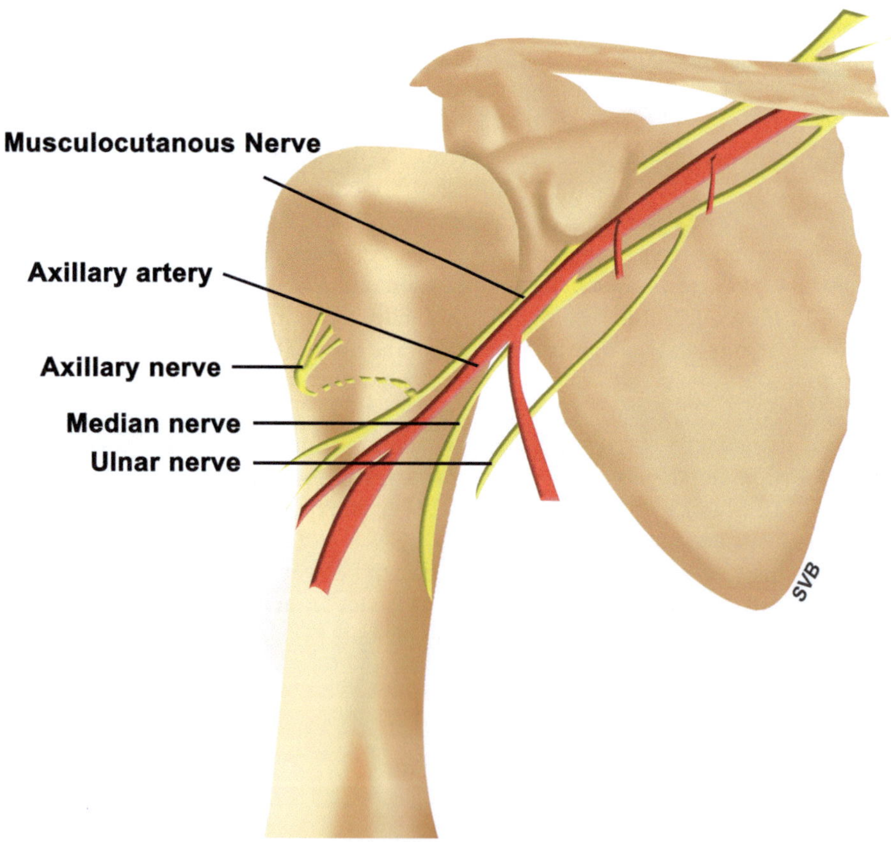

Fig. 3.1 The shoulder and its neurovascular relations

3.3 Principles of Safe Shoulder Surgery [2, 5–12]

3.3.1 Safety Principles for Approaching the Shoulder Joint Anteriorly

- The plane of dissection should be between the pectoralis major and the deltoid muscle.
- The axillary artery is surrounded by the cords of the brachial plexus, which lie just behind the pectoralis minor muscle. The second part of the axillary artery is inferior to the coracoid process underneath the pectoralis minor muscle. Abduction of the arm brings these vital structures close to the coracoid and the operative site. Hence, the arm should always be fully adducted during the surgery.
- Externally rotating the humerus increases the distance between the subscapularis muscle and the axillary nerve.
- The musculocutaneous nerve enters the belly of coracobrachialis about 5–8 cm distal to the muscle's origin at the coracoid process. Because the nerve enters the muscle from its medial side, all dissection must remain on the lateral side of the muscle. Utmost care to be taken not to retract the muscle inferiorly in order to avoid stretching of the nerve, which can lead to palsy of the elbow flexors.
- The cephalic vein should be preserved. However, a traumatized vein should be ligated to prevent any risk of thromboembolism.
- During coracoid osteotomy, if a screw is to be used, the coracoid process should be predrilled and tapped before commencing osteotomy.

3.3.2 Safety Principles for Approaching the Acromioclavicular Joint and Subacromial Space Anterolaterally

- The axillary nerve runs in a transverse direction, crossing the deep portion of the deltoid muscle about 7 cm below the tip of the acromion. Splitting the deltoid below this region will damage the nerve. Insert a stay suture in the apex of the deltoid split to safeguard the nerve.
- Care must be taken during surgical dissection in this approach not to damage the acromial branch of the coracoacromial artery that runs just under the deltoid muscle.

3.3.3 Safety Principles for the Lateral Approach to the Proximal Humerus

- The axillary nerve leaves the posterior wall of the axilla by passing through the quadrangular space. Then it winds around the humerus along, with the posterior circumflex humeral arteries. The nerve enters the deltoid muscle posteriorly from its deeper region, approximately 7 cm inferior to the tip of the acromion.

3.3.4 Safety Principles for Accessing the Proximal Humerus by the Minimal Lateral Approach

- This approach is through two incisions. Again, the axillary nerve has to be carefully guarded. It runs along the underside of the deltoid. As long as the surgeon operates underneath the deltoid muscle and on the bone, the nerve will not be injured.
- Do not forcefully retract the deltoid muscle fibers in any direction, as this may injure the axillary nerve.

3.3.5 Safety Principles for Approaching the Shoulder Joint Posteriorly

- The axillary nerve runs through the quadrangular space inferior to the teres minor muscle. The dissection plane should be in the space between the teres minor and the infraspinatus. The suprascapular nerve runs around the base of the spine of the scapula as it goes from the supraspinous fossa to the infraspinous fossa. It supplies both the supraspinatus and infraspinatus muscles. The infraspinatus should not be retracted vigorously too far medially during this approach because a neuropraxia can result from stretching the nerve on the lateral edge of the scapular spine.
- The posterior circumflex humeral artery runs with the axillary nerve in the quadrangular space beneath the lower border of the teres minor muscle. Damage to this artery leads to hemorrhage that will be difficult to control. This risk can be safely prevented by staying in the correct intermuscular plane

3.3.6 Safety Principles for Arthroscopic Shoulder Surgery

- Correct arthroscopic portal placement is essential in shoulder arthroscopy. The main portal sites are posterior (2 cm below and medial to the posterolateral corner of the acromion) and lateral (1–2 cm posterior, 2–3 cm lateral to the anterolateral corner of the acromion).
- The axillary nerve runs to the posterior wall of the axilla by passing the quadrangular space. It courses around the humerus, following the deep region of the deltoid muscle approximately 7 cm below the tip of the acromion. If the posterior portal is properly located in relation to posterolateral tip of the acromion, it will be about 3 cm superior to the nerve. Only a very inferiorly and incorrectly placed incision will endanger the nerve.
- The suprascapular nerve runs around the base of the spine of the scapula as it passes from the supraspinatus fossa to the infraspinatus fossa. This nerve is in danger if the posterior portal is made too medially. The correct portal position is 2 cm lateral to the nerve.

- The axillary nerve may be at risk from superiorly placed incisions as it traverses along the deeper surface of the deltoid muscle.
- The musculocutaneous nerve, which supplies flexor muscles of the upper arm, enters those muscles approximately 2–8 cm distal to the tip of the coracoids process. Thus, the nerve is unlikely to be damaged by a portal made superior and lateral to the level of the coracoid process.

3.4 Discussion

Locking plate and screw systems present a noteworthy treatment option in the management of complex and displaced humerus fractures. A precise indication, protection of the humeral head's inclination angle through correct surgical approach and technique, and fine calculation of screw length are important for successful functional results [9].

Deep infection with *Propionibacterium acnes* has been reported following shoulder arthroscopy, and the shoulder surgeon should have an high index of suspicion to tackle this situation effectively [1]. Implementation of an antibiotic stewardship program and safety protocols in all the health establishments is highly recommended to prevent and manage surgical site infections [13–17] (see also Chap. 1).

References

1. Moen TC, Rudolph GH, Caswell K et al (2014) Complications of shoulder arthroscopy. J Am Acad Orthop Surg 22(7):410–419
2. Weber SC, Abrams JS, Nottage WM (2002) Complications associated with arthroscopic shoulder surgery. Arthroscopy 18(2 Suppl 1):88–95
3. Shin JJ, Popchak AJ, Musahl V et al (2018) Complications after arthroscopic shoulder surgery: a review of the American Board of Orthopaedic Surgery Database. J Am Acad Orthop Surg Glob Res Rev 2(12):e093
4. Klug A, Wincheringer D, Harth J et al (2019) Complications after surgical treatment of proximal humerus fractures in the elderly: an analysis of complication patterns and risk factors for reverse shoulder arthroplasty and angular-stable plating. J Shoulder Elbow Surg 28(9):1674–1684
5. Boardman ND 3rd, Cofield RH (1999) Neurologic complications of shoulder surgery. Clin Orthop Relat Res 368:44–53
6. Beecroft CL, Coventry DM (2008) Anaesthesia for shoulder surgery. Contin Educ Anaesth Crit Care Pain 8(6):193–198
7. Depalma AF (2008) Surgical anatomy of the rotator cuff and the natural history of degenerative periarthritis. Clin Orthop Relat Res 466:543–551
8. Hoppenfeld S, de Boer P, Buckley R (2022) Surgical exposures in orthopaedics: the anatomic approach, 6th edn. Wolters Kluwer, Philadelphia
9. Aksu N, Göğüş A, Kara AN, Işiklar ZU (2010) Complications encountered in proximal humerus fractures treated with locking plate fixation. Acta Orthop Traumatol Turc 44(2):89–96
10. Millett PJ, van der Meijden OAJ, Gaskill T (2012) Surgical anatomy of the shoulder. Instr Course Lect 61:87–95
11. Eichinger JK, Galvin JW (2015) Management of complications after total shoulder arthroplasty. Curr Rev Musculoskelet Med 8(1):83–91

12. Gregory TM, Boukebous B, Gregory J et al (2017) Short, medium and long term complications after total anatomical shoulder arthroplasty. Open Orthop J 11:1133–1141
13. World Alliance for Patient Safety (2009) Safe surgery saves lives: the second global safety challenge. World Health Organization website. https://www.who.int/patientsafety/safesurgery/knowledge_base/SSSL_Brochure_finalJun08.pdf
14. World Health Organization (2019) Antimicrobial stewardship programmes in health-care facilities in low- and middle-income countries: a WHO practical toolkit. https://www.who.int/publications/i/item/9789241515481
15. National Institute for Health and Care Excellence (2015, August 18) Antimicrobial stewardship: systems and processes for effective antimicrobial medicine use. NICE guideline 15. https://www.nice.org.uk/guidance/ng15
16. National Institute for Health and Care Excellence (2019) Surgical site infections: prevention and treatment. NICE guideline 125. https://www.nice.org.uk/guidance/ng125
17. Seligman KM, Katz D, Farber MK (2018) Preventing surgical site infection after cesarean delivery: the anesthesia professional's role. APSF Newsl 33(1):25–27

Safe Humerus Surgery

4

4.1 Introduction

The incidence of humeral shaft fractures is about 5% of all fractures [1]. They occur almost entirely as a result of high-energy trauma in young individuals or following low-energy trauma in the elderly.

Classically, the treatment of humeral diaphyseal fractures has been conservative, but the morbidity and related consequences, as well as a lower tolerance for residual deformity, have led to a greater indication for surgical treatment in recent years [2]. The increase in surgical treatment of humeral shaft fractures has come at the cost of a higher risk of complications. All surgeries around the humerus are potentially risky because the important neurovascular structures in this region run much closer to the bone than anywhere else in the body.

Operative correction of humeral fractures is generally of four types—open reduction and internal fixation (ORIF), minimally invasive plate osteosynthesis (MIPO), intramedullary nailing, and external fixation [2]. If the fracture is open, significantly displaced, or associated with a neurovascular injury, it requires definite surgical treatment with exploration of the vital structures. MIPO and anterograde or retrograde locked intramedullary nailing require precise skills and instrumentation, as well as good knowledge of the pertinent anatomy to avoid complications associated with the techniques [1].

4.2 Applied Surgical Anatomy of the Humerus and Arm [3–9]

The surgeon must possess the detailed anatomic understanding of orthopaedic surgical approaches and precise skills for safe surgery (Fig. 4.1).

Numerous muscles have insertions on the humerus, which can displace fracture fragments. The medullary cavity is funnel shaped. The proximal segment has a

S. V. Babu, *Safe Orthopaedic Surgery*,
https://doi.org/10.1007/978-981-16-2846-7_4

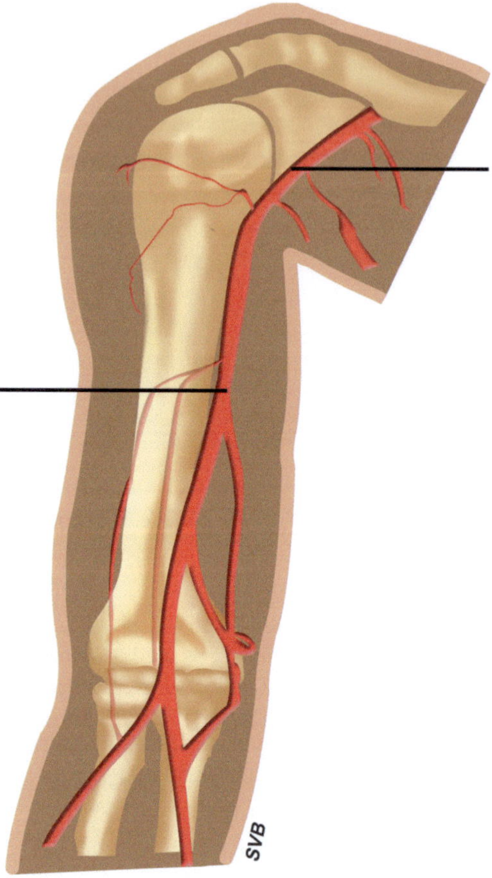

Fig. 4.1 The humerus and its vascular relations

larger diameter and relatively round. The distal segment is flatter and has a smaller diameter. This segment has an elongated S-shape in the oblique posterior and medial planes, which corresponds to the humeral head's retroversion axis. The axial torsion in the humeral diaphysis results in two smooth surfaces: one is the longer anteromedial portion and the other is the shorter anterolateral one (the region through which the radial nerve passes).

The axillary, radial, and ulnar nerves are directly related to the humerus, the radial being at greatest risk during exposure of the humeral shaft. A clear understand of the structural relationship of the humerus with these nerves is vital during surgery in this region.

- The **radial nerve** is in close apposition to the posterior portion of the shaft of the humerus. This is the reason for the higher number of primary palsy cases. The nerve runs in an oblique posterior groove from internal to external and superior to inferior over 6.5 cm. It runs on the lateral intermuscular septum at 16 cm from

the lateral humeral epicondyle, which makes it vulnerable to displaced humeral fractures, particularly at the junction between the middle and lower thirds. Individual dissimilarity in the crossing point results in a "risk/danger area" 10–15 cm from the lateral epicondyle of the humerus. The exact position of the radial was had been defined in a cadaver study: it comes into contact with the posterior side of the humerus at 20.7 ± 1.2 cm from the medial epicondyle and leaves it 14.2 ± 0.6 cm from the medial epicondyle.
- The **axillary nerve** runs around the posterior side of the surgical neck from internal to external, while following a horizontal arc 45 mm below the greater tuberosity of the humerus. It is flattened against the posterior side of the humerus.
- The **ulnar nerve** is located just behind the medial septum. It is near the posteromedial border of the distal segment of the humerus, where it can be damaged during the surgical approach or when using instruments.

The vascularization of the humeral diaphysis is heterogenous. It is very low in the distal third, which explains the greater number of nonunions at this level.

The humerus is directed mostly by rotational and distraction forces; it is not subjected to compressive forces. The chosen fixation method should neutralize all the rotational forces to achieve union by first modality.

4.3 Safe Principles of Humerus Surgery [1, 3, 7, 10–21]

Requirements for safe surgery include marking the surgical site with precise identification of the plane and neurovascular structures, as well as proper patient positioning. A supportive anaesthetist colleague who is able to effectively manage the patient's physiologic factors is important. Guidelines should be followed to prevent surgical site infection.

4.3.1 Safety Principles for the Anterior Approach to the Humeral Shaft

- The radial nerve is risk at two places:
  - At the spiral groove, posterior of the middle third of the humerus. It can be injured by drills, taps, and bone screws that are inserted anteroposteriorly when anterior plates are being applied in the middle third of the bone.
  - In the anterior compartment of the distal third of the arm, where the nerve pierces the lateral intermuscular septum and lies between the brachioradialis and brachialis muscles. It must be borne in mind that this plane is oblique and not vertical. To protect the nerve, the brachialis must be split along its midline.
- The axillary nerve, which runs under the deltoid muscle, can be damaged as a result of a compression injury caused by overly forceful retraction of the muscle. Extreme care must be taken when placing retractors on the deltoid to avoid injuring the nerve.

- The anterior circumflex humeral vessels cross the operative field in the interval between the pectoralis major muscle and deltoid in the upper third of the arm. They should be ligated or diathermized rather than cut with a scalpel.

4.3.2 Safety Principles for the Minimally Invasive Anterior Approach to the Humeral Shaft

- The two-incision minimally invasive approach uses a 5–7-cm longitudinal incision beginning just below the coracoid process and running down the arm in the line of the deltopectoral groove. Then a 5–7-cm longitudinal second incision is made over the lateral border of the biceps brachii muscle in the distal third of the arm.
  - The radial nerve runs lateral to this surgical approach in the distal window, lying between the lateral border of the brachialis and the brachioradialis.
- The muscular cutaneous nerve and its distal branch, the lateral antebrachial cutaneous nerve, lie medial to the brachialis and the distal window. To protect these two nerves, the brachialis has to be split in its midline.
- The anterior circumflex humeral vessels cross the operative field as explained earlier, in the interval between the pectoralis major and the deltoid muscle in the upper third of the arm. These vital structures have to be identified during development of the submuscular plane, and utmost care is warranted.

4.3.3 Safety Principles for the Anterolateral Approach to the Distal Humerus

- The radial nerve has to be identified and preserved before any incision is made through the belly of the brachialis muscle.

4.3.4 Safety Principles for the Posterior Approach to the Distal Humerus

- The radial nerve is at risk in the spiral groove. After it is identified, the dissection should never be continued down to bone in the proximal two thirds of the arm.

4.3.5 Safety Principles for the Lateral Approach to the Distal Humerus

- The radial nerve runs through the lateral intermuscular septum in the distal third of the arm. It is safe as long as the approach is not extended proximally

4.3.6 Safety Principles for the Minimally Invasive Approach for Humeral Nailing

- The axillary nerve is about 7 cm inferior to the tip of the acromion, running transversely on the deep region of the deltoid muscle. The nerve can be damaged by proximal interlocking bolts inserted from lateral to medial side.
- The brachial artery and median nerve lie just medial to the proximal humerus. They are also in danger during insertion of proximal locking screws.

4.3.7 Safety Principles for External Fixation of the Humerus

- The bicortical pins should be inserted on the lateral side of the humerus under image intensifier control, keeping the nerve relations well in mind.
- The proximal pins must be inserted distally to the axillary nerve; the distal pins must avoid the "danger/risk area" associated with the radial nerve, as explained before.

4.4 Discussion

While humeral shaft fractures are often treated conservatively, the combination of the progress that has been made with internal fixation devices and pressure from patients has led to increased use of surgical management. Although the bone union is faster in conservative treatment (9 weeks) than in surgical fixation (11–19 weeks), as is functional recovery, surgical treatment of humerus fractures is preferred today [1].

ORIF is associated with anatomic reduction but also with operative complications such as infection, fixation failure, secondary radial nerve palsy and nonunion [1]. However, MIPO is well accepted and recommended for both simple and complex humeral shaft fractures [9, 12, 13, 15, 18, 19, 22–26].

It is highly recommended that all health establishments implement an antibiotic stewardship program and safety protocols to prevent and manage surgical site infections [14, 17, 20, 27, 28] (see also Chap. 1).

References

1. Pidhorz L (2015) Acute and chronic humeral shaft fractures in adults. Orthop Traumatol Surg Res 101(1 suppl):S41–S49
2. Gonçalves FF, Dau L, Grassi CA et al (2018) Evaluation of the surgical treatment of humeral shaft fractures and comparison between surgical fixation methods. Rev Bras Ortop 53(2):136–141
3. Hoppenfeld S, de Boer P, Buckley R (2021) Surgical exposures in orthopaedics: the anatomic approach, 6th edn. Wolters Kluwer, Philadelphia

4. Hofman M, Grommes J, Krombach GA, Schmidt-Rohlfing B (2011) Vascular injury accompanying displaced proximal humeral fractures: two cases and a review of the literature. Emerg Med Int 2011:742870
5. Kumar V, Behera P, Aggarwal S, Kumar MU (2013) Iatrogenic brachial artery injury during anterolateral plating of humeral shaft fracture. Chin J Traumatol 16(6):371–374
6. Bichsel U, Nyffeler RW (2015) Secondary radial nerve palsy after minimally invasive plate osteosynthesis of a distal humeral shaft fracture. Case Rep Orthop 2015:241968
7. Belayneh R, Lott A, Haglin J et al (2019) Final outcomes of radial nerve palsy associated with humeral shaft fracture and nonunion. J Orthop Traumatol 20(1):18
8. Bounds EJ, Frane N, Kok SJ (2021) Humeral shaft fractures. In: StatPearls. StatPearls Publishing, Treasure Island, FL. https://www.ncbi.nlm.nih.gov/books/NBK448074/
9. Sharma B, Metia S, Kapoor K, Poswal P (2018) Delayed presentation of brachial artery injury following fracture shaft humerus; whether amputate or salvage: a series of two cases. J Orthop Traumatol Rehabil 10(2):137–141
10. Gainor BJ, Metzler M (1986) Humeral shaft fracture with brachial artery injury. Clin Orthop Relat Res 204:154–161
11. Lin J, Shen P-W, Hou S-M (2003) Complications of locked nailing in humeral shaft fractures. J Trauma 54(5):943–949
12. Jiang R, Luo C-F, Zeng B-F, Mei G-H (2007) Minimally invasive plating for complex humeral shaft fractures. Arch Orthop Trauma Surg 127(7):531–535
13. An Z, Zeng B-F, Wang Y et al (2007) Minimally invasive plating osteosynthesis (MIPO) of middle and distal third humeral shaft fractures. J Orthop Trauma 21(9):628–633
14. World Health Organization (2009) WHO guidelines for safe surgery: safe surgery saves lives. https://www.who.int/teams/integrated-health-services/patient-safety/research/safe-surgery&publication=9789241598552
15. Spagnolo R, Pace F, Bonalumi M (2010) Minimally invasive plating osteosynthesis technique applied to humeral shaft fractures: the lateral approach. Eur J Orthop Traumatol 20:205–210
16. Wang C, Li J, Li Y et al (2015) Is minimally invasive plating osteosynthesis for humeral shaft fracture advantageous compared with the conventional open technique? J Shoulder Elbow Surg 24(11):1741–1748
17. National Institute for Health and Care Excellence (2015, August 18) Antimicrobial stewardship: systems and processes for effective antimicrobial medicine use. NICE guideline 15. https://www.nice.org.uk/guidance/ng15
18. Kim JW, Oh C-W, Byun Y-S et al (2015) A prospective randomized study of operative treatment for noncomminuted humeral shaft fractures: conventional open plating versus minimal invasive plate osteosynthesis. J Orthop Trauma 29(4):189–194
19. Lee T, Yoon J (2016) Newly designed minimally invasive plating of a humerus shaft fracture; a different introduction of the plate. Int Orthop 40(12):2597–2602
20. Seligman KM, Katz D, Farber MK (2018) Preventing surgical site infection after cesarean delivery: the anesthesia professional's role. APSF Newsl 33(1):25–27
21. Schwab TR, Stillhard PF, Schibli S et al (2018) Radial nerve palsy in humeral shaft fractures with internal fixation: analysis of management and outcome. Eur J Trauma Emerg Surg 44(2):232–243
22. Oh C-W, Byun Y-S, Oh J-K et al (2012) Plating of humeral shaft fractures: comparison of standard conventional plating versus minimally invasive plating. Orthop Traumatol Surg Res 98(1):54–60
23. Hu X, Xu S, Lu H et al (2016) Minimally invasive plate osteosynthesis vs conventional fixation techniques for surgically treated humeral shaft fractures: a meta analysis. J Orthop Surg Res 11:59
24. Zhao J-G, Wang J, Huang W-J, Zhang P (2019) Surgical interventions for treating humeral shaft fractures in adults. Cochrane Database Syst Rev 2019(5):CD012174
25. Tetsworth K, Hohmann E, Glatt V (2018) Minimally invasive plate osteosynthesis of humeral shaft fractures: current state of the art. J Am Acad Orthop Surg 26(18):652–661

26. Lal YM, Mishra AK, Kushwaha AS, Badoni N (2019) A clinical study of anterior bridge plating for humerus shaft fractures by minimal invasive technique. Int J Orthop Sci 5(3):122–125
27. World Health Organization (2019) Antimicrobial stewardship programmes in health-care facilities in low- and middle-income countries: a WHO practical toolkit. https://www.who.int/publications/i/item/9789241515481
28. National Institute for Health and Care Excellence (2019) Surgical site infections: prevention and treatment. NICE guideline 125. https://www.nice.org.uk/guidance/ng125

5 Safe Elbow Surgery

5.1 Introduction

The elbow is a trochoginglymoid joint, meaning the joint is a combination of hinge and pivot that permits movement in both flexion-extension and pronation-supination from all these articulations. Not surprisingly, fractures of the elbow can be technically demanding to treat, with significant complications [1].

Most elbow disorders and fractures are surgically treated one of three ways—openly, minimally invasively, or arthroscopically. During the past two decades, the use of arthroscopy in elbow surgery has increased dramatically. The propinquity of neurovascular structures and the narrow joint spaces make elbow arthroscopy technically challenging and subject to many potential complications, such as ulnar nerve injury, surgical site infections, and elbow contracture. But these technical hitches can be prevented when performed in a standardized fashion by experienced hands [2, 3].

Innovative advances in implant design and improvement of surgical techniques have stretched the applications of total elbow arthroplasty. Unfortunately, however, the complications associated with reconstructive elbow surgery can lead to profound and sometimes unsalvageable disability. The most frequently documented complications include implant loosening, periprosthetic fracture, implant failure, surgical site infection, triceps insufficiency, and nerve palsy. Although fewer elbow arthroplasties are performed than lower extremity arthroplasties, complication rates are higher with elbow arthroplasty and the outcomes of secondary reconstruction are less favorable [4–6].

Minimally invasive plate osteosynthesis (MIPO) techniques have been suggested for the treatment of comminuted fractures, because they encourage biologic fixation without devitalization of bone fragments [7]. MIPO has been extensively used in the management of fractures of the humerus with good results.

S. V. Babu, *Safe Orthopaedic Surgery*,
https://doi.org/10.1007/978-981-16-2846-7_5

5.2 Applied Surgical Anatomy of the Elbow

Knowledge of the surgical anatomy around the elbow, the neurovascular structures, and the surgical planes is imperative for to the performance of safe surgery. For example, in fractures of the distal third of humeral shaft, the radial nerve in this area has lower mobility and is closer to the bone. Thus, there is a greater possibility for iatrogenic nerve injury during fracture reduction [8].

Identifying nerves, veins, arteries, and other vital structures and understanding their relationships are key to operating effectively in the cubital fossa and the elbow joint (Fig. 5.1).

5.3 Principles of Safe Elbow Surgery [8–15]

5.3.1 Safety Principles for the Posterior Approach to Elbow Joint

- The ulnar nerve can be protected as long as it is identified early in the procedure. Dissect it free and pass colored material around it so that it can be safeguarded at all times. Excessive traction is to be avoided.
- The median nerve runs well anterior to the distal humerus. It can be at risk if the anterior structures are not dissected precisely from the distal humerus.
- The radial nerve is at risk if the surgery in the distal third of the humerus, especially above the lateral epicondylar region.
- The brachial artery runs along with the median nerve anteriorly in the elbow. It should be given the same protection as the nerve.

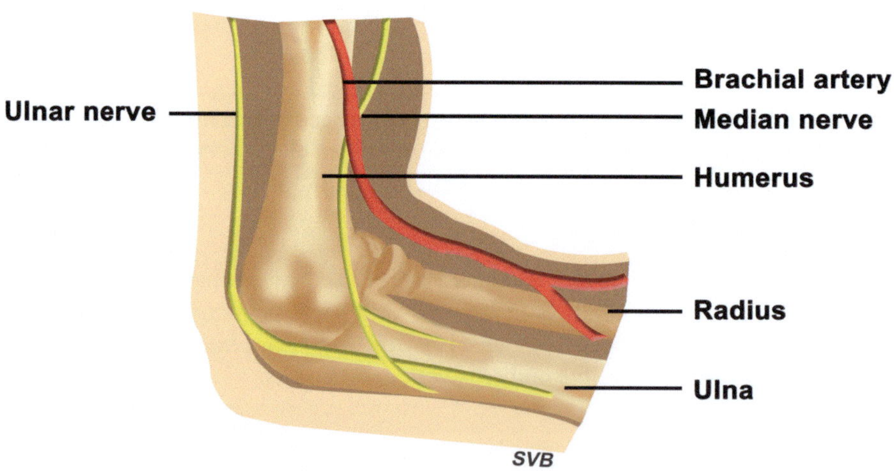

Fig. 5.1 The elbow and its neurovascular relations

5.3.2 Safety Principles for the Medial Approach to Elbow Joint

- Feel the ulnar nerve as it lies in its groove posteriorly in the medial condyle of the humerus. Carefully incise the fascia over the nerve starting proximal to the medial condyle, then the nerve can be separated along the incision.
- Establish the interval between the pronator teres and brachialis muscles, taking utmost care not to insult the median nerve, which passes through the pronator teres near the midline.
- Softly retract the pronator teres medially from the brachialis. Make sure the ulnar nerve is taken care of inferiorly, then carry out osteotomy of the medial epicondyle if it is needed.

5.3.3 Safety Principles for the Anterolateral Approach to the Elbow Joint

- First, recognize the lateral cutaneous nerve of the forearm (the sensory branch of the musculocutaneous nerve) as it becomes superficial to the deep fascia in the distal few centimeters of the arm just lateral to the biceps tendon in the interval between it and the brachialis muscle.
- Identify the radial nerve proximally at the level of the elbow joint in between the brachialis muscle and the brachioradialis muscle. The nerve runs anteromedial to the brachioradialis and crosses in front of elbow joint.
- The posterior interosseous nerve is in danger as it runs around the neck of the radius within the muscle belly of the supinator muscle. To prevent damage to the nerve, make sure that the forearm is in supination when the supinator is dissected from its insertion on the radius.
- Recognize the radial artery as it runs deep to the biceps tendon. Also identify its aponeurosis proximally to its origin from the brachial artery. Both the brachial vein and the median nerve are medial to the brachial artery

5.3.4 Safety Principles for the Anterior Approach to the Cubital Fossa

- The lateral cutaneous nerve of the forearm to be protected. To identify it, go to the space between the biceps tendon and the brachialis muscle; the nerve emerges there to pass down the lateral region of the forearm in the subcutaneous plane.
- Be careful not to injure the brachial artery, which runs immediately under the bicipital aponeurosis.

5.3.5 Safety Principles for the Posterolateral Approach to the Radial Head

- The radial nerve is protected when the elbow joint is opened laterally and not anteriorly.
- The posterior interosseous nerve is protected when the dissection remains proximal to the annular ligament. Pronation of the forearm keeps the nerve at distance from the operative field.

5.3.6 Safety Principles for Arthroscopic Elbow Surgery

- The proximal anteromedial portal is created first, approximately 2 cm proximal to the medial epicondyle and anterior to the intermuscular septum. Always stay anterior to the intermuscular septum, which protects the ulnar nerve, located 3–4 mm from this portal. The nerve is identified by blunt dissection through this portal until the anterior surface of humerus bone is palpated. This is the significant step. If the portal is placed too anterior, the neurovascular structures in the cubital fossa (the median nerve and the brachial artery) are in danger. If the portal is made posterior to the humerus, also posterior to the intermuscular septum, the ulnar nerve can be damaged.
- Next, the anterolateral portal is made by an out–in technique. It is created 2 cm proximal and 1 cm anterior to the lateral epicondyle. If this portal is placed too far distally, near to the radial neck, the posterior interosseous nerve can be damaged.
- For examining the posterior compartment, a straight posterior portal is regularly established first, 3 cm proximal to the tip of the olecranon. This portal passes within 25 mm of the ulnar nerve and within 23 mm of the posterior cutaneous nerve of forearm. Take care to dissect the ulnar nerve free to avoid injury [12, 13].
- Then the posterolateral portal is placed 2–3 cm proximal to the tip of olecranon at the lateral surface of the triceps tendon. The medial and posterior cutaneous nerves of the forearm run an average of 25 mm from this portal, placing them at risk. The ulnar nerve may be injured near the medial epicondyle and the medial gutter.
- The lateral portal is created at the "soft spot"—the triangle formed by the radial head, lateral epicondyle, and olecranon.

5.3.7 Safety Principles for the Minimally Invasive Approach to the Elbow Joint

- For MIPO of distal humerus, proximal access is created between the tendon of the biceps muscle medially and the tendon of the deltoid muscle and the cephalic vein laterally. Next, the arm is abducted around 60° and 90° to correct the typical varus deviation. Then the plate is introduced proximally to distally.

- After the plate is placed on the anterior surface of humeral diaphysis, the mean distance from the closest part of the plate to the radial nerve is 3.2 mm. When a plate is inserted submuscularly through two small incisions on the anterior side of the arm away from the fracture site, the brachial muscle covers most of the anteriorly placed plate and protects the radial nerve from injury.

5.4 Discussion

Total elbow arthroplasty is a feasible choice for advanced degenerative disease of the elbow. Good pain relief and reestablishment of function have broadened surgical indications to include complex fractures of the distal humerus, joint ankylosis, and severe elbow instability. Satisfactory outcomes can be expected in more than 75% of patients, but the rates of aseptic and septic complications and revision surgeries remain high [4].

Elbow arthroscopy is a relatively safe procedure and is used increasingly to treat complex pathology. In less experienced hands, however, it can lead to more complications, including infections and neurologic injuries [3, 5, 11].

The radial head has been increasingly recognized as an significant stabilizer of the elbow. Radial head fractures may have associated elbow dislocation, coronoid process fractures, ulnar fractures, capitellar injuries, and rupture of interosseous membrane. The main aim in the treatment of radial head fractures is to reinstate the anatomy of the radial head and surrounding tissues to achieve a stable and functional elbow joint, a goal that justifies surgical management [16].

Over the past two decades, a higher incidence of complex fractures of the distal humerus has been seen as a result of injuries caused by high-energy trauma [7, 10, 14]. Surgical treatment is necessary for these fractures, considering the articular involvement and to retain the biomechanics of the elbow joint. MIPO shows potential when compared with conventional plating and nailing in distal humerus fractures. MIPO has advantages in terms of a lower incidence of iatrogenic radial nerve injuries and also in faster fracture union and a likely functional outcome with respect to shoulder and elbow function [7, 10, 14].

It is highly recommended that all health establishments implement an antibiotic stewardship program and safety protocols to prevent and manage surgical site infections [17–21] (see also Chap. 1).

References

1. Cheung EV, Sarkissian EJ (2015) Complications of elbow trauma. Hand Clin 31(4):683–691
2. Kelly EW, Morrey BF, O'Driscoll SW (2001) Complications of elbow arthroscopy. J Bone Joint Surg Am 83(1):25–34
3. Elfeddali R, Schreuder MHE, Eygendaal D (2013) Arthroscopic elbow surgery: is it safe? J Shoulder Elbow Surg 22(5):647–652
4. Kim JM, Mudgal CS, Konopka JF, Jupiter JB (2011) Complications of total elbow arthroplasty. J Am Acad Orthop Surg 19(6):328–339

5. Nelson GN, Wu T, Galatz LM et al (2014) Elbow arthroscopy: early complications and associated risk factors. J Shoulder Elbow Surg 23(2):273–278
6. Ornell SS, Dang KH, Bois AJ, Dutta AK (2019) Fungal infection following total elbow arthroplasty. Case Rep Orthop 2019:7927914
7. Zogaib RK, Morgan S, Belangero PS et al (2014) Minimal invasive ostheosintesis for treatment of diaphiseal transverse humeral shaft fractures. Acta Ortop Bras 22(2):94–98
8. Zogbi DR, Terrivel AM, Mouraria GG et al (2014) Fracture of distal humerus: MIPO technique with visualization of the radial nerve. Acta Orthop Bras 22(6):300–303
9. Hoppenfeld S, de Boer P, Buckley R (2022) Surgical exposures in orthopaedics: the anatomic approach, 6th edn. Wolters Kluwer, Philadelphia
10. An Z, Zeng B, He X et al (2010) Plating osteosynthesis of mid-distal humeral shaft fractures: minimally invasive versus conventional open reduction technique. Int Orthop 34(1):131–135
11. Mardani-Kivi M, Kazemnejad E, Hashemi-Motlagh K, Saheb-Ekhtiari K (2018) Indications, results and complications of elbow arthroscopy treatment in eighteen patients. Shiraz E-Med J 19(6):e62606
12. Stetson WB, Vogeli K, Chung B et al (2018) Avoiding neurological complications of elbow arthroscopy. Arthrosc Tech 7(7):e717–e724
13. Stetson WB, Vogeli K, Chung B et al (2018) Neurological complications of elbow arthroscopy. In: Amarasekera HW (ed) Recent advances in arthroscopic surgery, IntechOpen book series. IntechOpen, London, p 639
14. Savvidou OD, Zampeli F, Koutsouradis P et al (2018) Complications of open reduction and internal fixation of distal humerus fractures. EFORT Open Rev 3(10):558–567
15. Kwak J-M, Koh K-H, Jeon I-H (2019) Total elbow arthroplasty: clinical outcomes, complications, and revision surgery. Clin Orthop Surg 11(4):369–379
16. Kodde IF, Kaas L, Flipsen M et al (2015) Current concepts in the management of radial head fractures. World J Orthop 6(11):954–960
17. World Alliance for Patient Safety (2009) Safe surgery saves lives: the second global safety challenge. World Health Organization website. https://www.who.int/patientsafety/safesurgery/knowledge_base/SSSL_Brochure_finalJun08.pdf
18. World Health Organization (2019) Antimicrobial stewardship programmes in health-care facilities in low- and middle-income countries: a WHO practical toolkit. https://www.who.int/publications/i/item/9789241515481
19. National Institute for Health and Care Excellence (2015, August 18) Antimicrobial stewardship: systems and processes for effective antimicrobial medicine use. NICE guideline 15. https://www.nice.org.uk/guidance/ng15
20. National Institute for Health and Care Excellence (2019) Surgical site infections: prevention and treatment. NICE guideline 125. https://www.nice.org.uk/guidance/ng125
21. Seligman KM, Katz D, Farber MK (2018) Preventing surgical site infection after cesarean delivery: the anesthesia professional's role. APSF Newsl 33(1):25–27

6 Safe Forearm Surgery

6.1 Introduction

The forearm has a multifarious anatomy that comprises the radius, the ulna, and their intraosseous membranes well surrounded by muscles and close neurovascular structures. The supination and pronation movements of the forearm originate from the proximal and distal radioulnar joints. Hence, the radius and ulna have a vital role in the movements of the forearm and also in the whole of upper extremity. Because of the bones' unique functional and anatomic features, forearm diaphyseal fractures are different from diaphyseal fractures of other long bones. These fractures should be evaluated as intra-articular fractures with management planned accordingly [1].

Open reduction and internal fixation (ORIF) with plate osteosynthesis, closed reduction with intramedullary locked nailing, external fixation, and elastic flexible nailing are the available surgical treatment choices. The primary goal of surgical fixation of forearm, either by an internal or external method, is to maintain length and alignment and to ensure there is no rotation of the fracture [2]. Inappropriate treatment of these fractures significantly affects total upper limb function as well as forearm function.

The surgical management of forearm fractures has been standardized except for children below the age of 10 years. The current established treatment is either plate osteosynthesis or elastic flexible nailing, each technique with its own advantages and disadvantages [1]. Based on functional and radiographic outcomes, the two techniques are similarly successful for forearm diaphyseal fractures management in early and mid-adolescent patients [3]. They also have a similar rate of neurovascular complications [4]. Plate fixation can have a high complication rate unless meticulous attention is paid to surgical technique [5, 6].

External fixation may be advocated for severe open fractures or in unstable polytraumatized patients for whom longer operations can be dangerous in damage-control orthopaedics [2, 7].

S. V. Babu, *Safe Orthopaedic Surgery*,
https://doi.org/10.1007/978-981-16-2846-7_6

6.2 Applied Surgical Anatomy of the Forearm

The two bones in the forearm have considerably different anatomy. The ulna has a full subcutaneous border that runs its entire length; thus, the bone can be reached simply and directly without disturbing other structures. But the upper two-thirds of the radius is fully enclosed by muscles. All surgeries in the upper third of the radius risk injuring the posterior interosseous nerve, which runs spirally around the bone [8] (Fig. 6.1).

Forearm fractures may be complicated by the disruption of the distal radioulnar, proximal radioulnar, or radiocapitellar joint. An important principle in managing fractures in this distinctive region injury is early acknowledgment and treatment of the injury. Maintaining length and reestablishing and preserving the anatomic axial and rotational alignment and the radial bow are all important in achieving satisfactory functional results and preserving range of motion [1, 9–11].

6.3 Principles of Safe Forearm Surgery [1–4, 6–10, 12–18]

6.3.1 Safety Principles for the Anterior Approach to the Radius

- In the proximal forearm, the median nerve typically runs in between the heads of the pronator teres muscle.

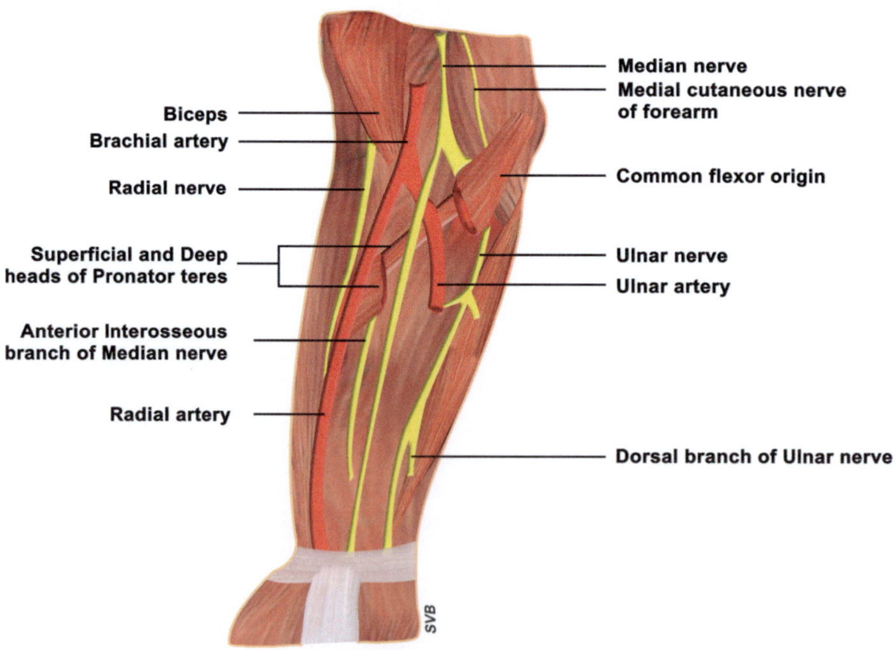

Fig. 6.1 The forearm and its neurovascular relations

- The posterior interosseous nerve is exposed as it runs around the neck of the radius within the muscle belly of the supinator. The principle to ensure its protection is to dissect accurately the insertion of the supinator from the radius. The insertion of the muscle is viewed only when the arm is completely supinated. When the subperiosteal dissection is started, the nerve is reasonably safe, but extensive retraction will lead to neuropraxia.
- The superficial radial nerve goes to the forearm underneath the brachioradialis muscle. It becomes exposed when the "mobile wad" of three muscles (brachioradialis, pronator teres, and flexor carpi radialis) is mobilized and retracted laterally. The superficial radial nerve is in danger of neuropraxia if it is pulled in forcefully.
- The radial artery runs in the center of the forearm inferior to the brachioradialis. It is at risk when approaching the radius anteriorly at two points:
  - First, during mobilization of the brachioradialis, utmost care must be taken to recognize the artery. The artery's two accompanying veins are the best surgical guide in avoiding injury.
  - Second, in the upper end of the wound, the radial artery runs to the medial side of the biceps tendon, so surgical dissection must remain lateral to the tendon to protect the artery here.
- The recurrent radial arteries are the branches of the radial artery that arise just below the elbow joint. They are in two groups, anterior and posterior, which pass in front of and behind the superficial radial nerve, before passing through the brachioradialis muscle. They must be ligated to allow mobilization of both the artery and the nerve.
- The ulnar artery runs deep to both heads of the pronator teres muscle.

6.3.2 Safety Principles for Exposure of the Shaft of the Ulna

- The ulnar nerve, which runs down the forearm just below the flexor carpi ulnaris, lies on the flexor digitorum profundus. The nerve is well protected as long as the flexor carpi ulnaris is not get dissected fully from the ulna.
- The ulnar artery travels to the forearm along with the ulnar nerve, lying on its radial side. It is safeguarded when dissection of the flexor carpi ulnaris is done subperiosteally.

6.3.3 Safety Principles for the Posterior Approach to the Radius

- The posterior interosseous nerve is in danger at two points:
  - First, while identifying the nerve. In about 25% of patients, the nerve actually lies on the dorsal aspect of the radius just across the bicipital tuberosity. If fixation plates are placed high on the dorsal region of the radius, they may injure the nerve below. The nerve must be carefully identified and preserved in the supinator muscle to protect it.

- Second, while saving the nerve with supinator muscle. The surgeon must dissect the supinator from the anterior surface of the radius and retract it laterally along with the nerve.

6.3.4 Safety Principles for External Fixation of Both Bones of the Forearm

- The modular external fixator is the most favorable for temporary use and sometimes as definite treatment in forearm fractures. It is quickly applied without need for intraoperative imaging and can be adjusted in the future.
- Two pins are inserted into each of the proximal and distal fragments at the safe zones. The risk of tendon penetration or injuries to nerves, vessels, and muscles is defined by the anatomy of each region. Pins should not be fixed where there is a possibility of entering a joint cavity.
- The anatomic relationships of the bones of the forearm are intricate because they depend on the rotational point of reference. For pin insertion, two forearm positions are most often used:
  - Pronation for the ulna
  - Neutral rotation (between pronation and supination) for the radius
- Safe zones for ulnar pin fixation are along the whole shaft of the bone between the extensor carpi ulnaris and the flexor carpi ulnaris muscles.
- The radial nerve is vulnerable in the proximal zone. The supinator muscle envelops the dorsal aspect of the upper third of the radius, with the posterior interosseous nerve running through its muscle belly.
- A skin incision is made and then gradually deepened by spreading forceps and advancing the retractors layer by layer until the bone is reached, then the application of the pin is carried out.
- In the distal zone of the radius, the surgeon must be aware of the superficial radial nerve and its muscles and extensor tendons. Any pins need to be fixed under direct vision using retractors down to the bone to avoid the superficial branch of the radial nerve.
- Pins are fixed on the dorsolateral aspect of the radius, just above Lister's tubercle in the muscle and tendon-free triangle between the tendons of the extensor carpi radialis brevis and extensor pollicis longus.

6.3.5 Safety Principles for Intramedullary Nailing of Both Bones of the Forearm

- An accurately sized nail has to be chosen carefully. If the selected nail's diameter is too large, it may produce an iatrogenic fracture; if the nail diameter is too small, it will lead to rotational instability.
- In radial nails, the proximal locking may lead to posterior interosseous nerve injury. The extensor pollicis longus tendon and superficial branch of the radial nerve are in danger at the wrist level entry point. Wider incision and precise dissection will prevent these entry point complications.

6.3.6 Safety Principles for Elastic Flexible Nailing of Both Bones of the Forearm in Children

- Universally, the radius will be the first to be operated on because it is easy to reduce.
- For the radius, the cortex at the point over the lateral aspect of the distal metaphysis, 2 cm proximal to the physis, has to be opened with a drill 1 mm larger than the size of the selected nail.
- For the ulna, it is advised to insert the pin through the proximal end, inferior to the olecranon apophysis, through an incision on the lateral aspect in relation to anconeus.

6.4 Discussion

Forearm fractures produce many unique challenges. The deforming force of the forearm muscles, permanence of the radial incline, and interosseous membrane injury are factors that affect the stabilization and preservation of fracture reduction. The best goal of surgical therapy is to provide axial alignment and rotational stability. The gold standard treatment for pediatric forearm fractures remains closed reduction and casting [19]. However, forearm fractures in older children treated with closed reduction and cast application have many complications and a failure rate of 11%, and these fractures necessitate revision surgery [3, 19]. Successful management of pediatric forearm fractures must produce painless and issueless outcomes with good purposeful pronation and supination. It has been reported that 15°–20° of angulation in middle-third forearm fractures will lead to a major reduction in forearm rotation [19]. The treating surgeon must keep this in mind to provide the best treatment possible [19].

Current consensus for both-bone forearm fractures surgery is that patients with malreduction with closed manipulation, open fractures, compartment syndrome, or ipsilateral humerus fractures causing a "floating elbow" should be managed with internal fixation. About 5% of all supracondylar humerus fractures in children have an ipsilateral forearm fracture as well. These fractures have significant risk of producing associated neurovascular injury, and the surgeon should carefully examine the preoperative neurovascular status of these patients [20].

Intramedullary nailing has advantages of smaller incision, shorter duration of anaesthesia and operating time, limited soft tissue injury, speedy union, and admirable recovery of movements over plate osteosynthesis [1, 3, 12]. Newly designed nails have proved successful in avoiding many complications. Open reduction and plating surgery produces a more anatomic fracture reduction, resulting in more accurate restoration of the radial bow, which is important for complete restoration of forearm rotation [1, 3, 12].

Hybrid fixation (plating of one bone and elastic nailing in the other) for adolescent both-bone diaphyseal forearm fractures has been reported to produce good stability and the best functional recovery outcomes [2, 4, 16, 21]. The risk of compartment syndrome can be increased, however, because of soft tissue trauma from repeated attempts of fracture reduction and intramedullary nail passage. Guidelines suggest a maximum of three intramedullary nail passing attempts to reduce the risk of compartment syndrome [14]. Refracture rates after forearm open reduction and internal fixation are significant, with the radius facing refracture more often than the ulna [22].

Intramedullary nailing of forearm fractures must be converted to open reduction in a significant proportion of cases [14]. A 10% incidence of superficial infections is associated with intramedullary nailing and around a 3% incidence of deep infection in plate osteosynthesis surgery [9–11]. There are many more complications in intramedullary nailing, which may be due to be either the surgeon's inexperience in the technique or the surgery itself [19].

Surgical management of pediatric forearm midshaft fractures by the orthopaedic specialist surgeons well trained in pediatric trauma offers advantages that include a shorter operating time and radiation time, and a minimal rate of open reduction in intramedullary nailing [13]. In general, severe comminution and bone loss should be considered as indications for plate fixation, though intramedullary nailing gives enhanced cosmesis and less soft tissue disruption [15].

Implementation of an antibiotic stewardship program and of safety protocols is recommended for all the health establishments to prevent and manage surgical site infections [18, 23–26].

References

1. Köse A, Aydin A, Ezirmik N, Yildirim ÖS (2017) A comparison of the treatment results of open reduction internal fixation and intramedullary nailing in adult forearm diaphyseal fractures. Ulus Travma Acil Cerrahi Derg 23(3):235–244
2. Hadeed A, Werntz RL, Varacallo M (2021) External fixation principles and overview. In: StatPearls. StatPearls Publishing, Treasure Island, FL. https://pubmed.ncbi.nlm.nih.gov/31613474/
3. Thapa UJ, Wahegaonkar K, Ranjeet N et al (2018) Comparative study in the outcome of intramedullary nailing to plating for both-bone forearm fracture in early and mid-adolescent age group. Med J DY Patil Vidyapeeth 11:499–505
4. Zhang XF, Huang JW, Mao HX et al (2016) Adult diaphyseal both-bone forearm fractures: a clinical and biomechanical comparison of four different fixations. Orthop Traumatol Surg Res 102(3):319–325
5. Stern PJ, Drury WJ (1983) Complications of plate fixation of forearm fractures. Clin Orthop Relat Res 175:25–29
6. Fernández Dell'Oca AA, Tepic S, Frigg R et al (2001) Treating forearm fractures using an internal fixator: a prospective study. Clin Orthop Relat Res 389:196–205
7. Mathieu L, Grosset A, Farah IH et al (2018) Temporary external fixation for forearm fractures in damage control orthopedics procedures: use of a simplified frame. Trauma Cases Rev 4(2):061
8. Hoppenfeld S, de Boer P, Buckley R (2022) Surgical exposures in orthopaedics: the anatomic approach, 6th edn. Wolters Kluwer, Philadelphia
9. Vishwanath C, Satheesh GS (2017) Surgical outcome of fracture both bones forearm in children using tens. Nat J Clin Orthop 1(2):16–23
10. Vishwanath C, Satheesh GS, Dwivedi S, Baruah M (2017) Surgical management of fracture both bones forearm in adults using LC-DCP. Int J Orthop Sci 3(1):97–108

11. Forsh DA, Cheung ZB (2021) Middle-third forearm fractures. Medscape Website. 1239870. http://emedicine.medscape.com/article/1239870
12. Köse A, Aydin A, Ezirmik N et al (2014) Alternate treatment of forearm double fractures: new design intramedullary nail. Arch Orthop Trauma Surg 134(10):1387–1396
13. Meena RK, Singh AM, Langshong R et al (2014) Internal fixation of adult diaphyseal both bone forearm fractures using locking compression plate. J Med Soc 28(3):171–174
14. Holt A, Snow EE, Shen K et al (2017) Risk factors for open reduction in operatively treated pediatric both-bone forearm fractures. OJHMS 18:14–19
15. Lu D, Lin Z, Zhang J-D et al (2017) Treatment of pediatric forearm midshaft fractures: is there a difference between types of orthopedic surgeon? Orthop Traumatol Surg Res 103(1):119–122
16. Chen C, Xie L, Zheng W et al (2019) Evaluating the safety and feasibility of a new surgical treatment for forearm fractures in older children: study protocol for a randomised controlled trial. Trials 20(1):320
17. Vem KB, Challa SK, Murthy D S (2019) Surgical management of fracture both bones forearm with locking compression plate in adult patients. Asian J Pharm Clin Res 12(3):130–135
18. World Health Organization (2019) Antimicrobial stewardship programmes in health-care facilities in low- and middle-income countries: a WHO practical toolkit. https://apps.who.int/iris/handle/10665/329404
19. Vopat ML, Kane PM, Christino MA et al (2014) Treatment of diaphyseal forearm fractures in children. Orthop Rev (Pavia) 6(2):5325
20. Muchow RD, Riccio AI, Garg S et al (2015) Neurological and vascular injury associated with supracondylar humerus fractures and ipsilateral forearm fractures in children. J Pediatr Orthop 35(2):121–125
21. Elhalawany AS, Afifi A, Anbar A, Galal S (2020) Hybrid fixation for adolescent both-bones diaphyseal forearm fractures: preliminary results of a prospective cohort study. J Clin Orthop Trauma 11(Suppl 1):S46–S50
22. Wolvetang N, Lans J, Chen NC (2018) Refractures after plate fixation of forearm fractures. J Hand Surg 43(9 Suppl):S24–S25
23. World Alliance for Patient Safety (2008) The second global safety challenge: safe surgery saves lives. World Health Organization website. https://www.who.int/patientsafety/safesurgery/knowledge_base/SSSL_Brochure_finalJun08.pdf
24. National Institute for Health and Care Excellence (2015) Antimicrobial stewardship: systems and processes for effective antimicrobial medicine use. NICE guideline 15. https://www.nice.org.uk/guidance/ng15
25. Seligman KM, Katz D, Farber MK (2018) Preventing surgical site infection after cesarean delivery: the anesthesia professional's role. APSF Newsl 33(1):25–27
26. National Institute for Health and Care Excellence (2020) Surgical site infections: prevention and treatment. NICE guideline 125. https://www.nice.org.uk/guidance/ng125

7 Safe Wrist and Hand Surgery

7.1 Introduction

Distal radius fractures are one of the most frequent fractures of the upper limb [1]. Surgical management is an excellent choice for displaced and unstable fractures. While current fixation techniques are effective, they are associated with many complications. Dorsal and volar plating, for example, are associated with tendon irritation and rupture, infection, and nerve injury. It is important for the surgeon to be aware of these complications and have treatment strategies to avoid them [1].

Nerve injury is a well-documented complication of upper limb orthopaedic surgery and may result from various causes. In hand and wrist surgery, the surgical incisions are small, which can make the course of small peripheral nerves difficult to identify and safeguard during retraction. Knowledge of potential neurologic and vascular complications will help the surgeon both during the procedure and in educating and counseling patients about perioperative risk. It will also assist in planning and in managing adverse events that may arise [2].

Wrist arthroscopy has increased in popularity to become the standard diagnostic procedure as well as a mainstay for treatment of pathologies of the wrist that it is today [3]. Although it has limitations, arthroscopy remains a valuable tool in investigating and treating wrist disorders. It is a safe surgery with a low rate of major and minor complications compared to arthroscopy of other joints [4].

Total wrist arthroplasty is an alternate for patients with severe wrist arthritis who are experiencing difficulties with activities of daily living. This surgery has its own specific risks and possible complications and is not advisable in patients with high physical demands [5].

S. V. Babu, *Safe Orthopaedic Surgery*,
https://doi.org/10.1007/978-981-16-2846-7_7

7.2 Applied Surgical Anatomy of the Hand and Wrist

The palmar aponeurosis is a strong fibrous sheath that lies under the skin of the palm. The nerves and vessels to the palm lie just below the aponeurosis and are in contact with its deep surface (Fig. 7.1). In patients with Dupuytren's contracture, the palmar fascia becomes thickened and contracted, and fibrous tissue grows around the digital nerves and vessels to capture them.

The flexor pollicis brevis of the thenar gets dual nerve supply from the median and ulnar nerves, especially to its deep head. Hence, full median nerve palsy does not necessarily flatten the thenar eminence. The abductor pollicis brevis is the key muscle in the eminence. Median nerve paralysis disrupts opposition, causing a simian (ape-like) hand.

The hypothenar eminence, including the palmaris brevis, is supplied by the ulnar nerve.

The second layer of the palm has the superficial nerves and vessels.

7.3 Principles of Safe Wrist and Hand Surgery [1, 2, 5–11]

7.3.1 Safety Principles for the Dorsal Approach to the Wrist Joint

- The radial nerve runs below the tendon of the brachioradialis muscle superior to the wrist joint before traveling to the dorsum of the hand. The surgeon has to identify and protect all the nerve branches that are encountered during incision of the subcutaneous tissue.
- The radial artery runs in the wrist on its lateral aspect. The dissection at the level of the wrist joint should remain well below the periosteum.

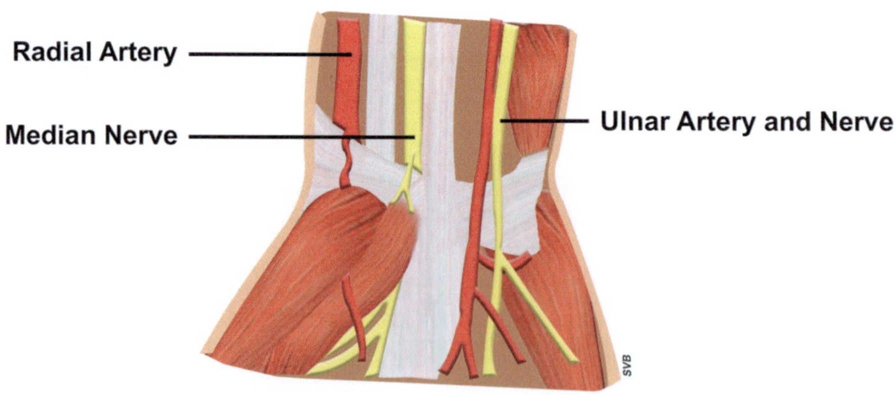

Fig. 7.1 The wrist and its neurovascular relations

7.3.2 Safety Principles for the Volar Approach to the Wrist Joint

- The palmar cutaneous branch of the median nerve branches out 5 cm proximal to the wrist joint and runs along the medial side of the tendon of the flexor carpi radialis muscle prior to crossing over the flexor retinaculum. The greatest danger to this nerve occurs if the skin incision is not acutely angled toward the medial side of the forearm.
- The motor branch of the median nerve to the thenar muscles exhibits significant anatomic variation. Threat to the nerve is minimized if the incision is done at the carpal tunnel on the medial side of the median nerve.
- The superficial palmar vascular arch crosses the palm at the level of the distal end of the outstretched thumb. The arch will be safe if the flexor retinaculum is divided cautiously under direct vision for its entire length.

7.3.3 Safety Principles for the Volar Approach to the Ulnar Nerve

- The ulnar nerve is exposed during two phases of the dissection—when the fascia on the lateral side of the flexor carpi ulnaris is incised to permit retraction of the muscle during superficial surgical dissection, and when volar carpal ligament is divided during deep surgical dissection.

7.3.4 Safety Principles for the Volar Approach to the Flexor Tendons

- The digital nerves and vessels can be injured if the skin mobilization extends too far in a dorsal direction.
- Skin flaps should not be incised as acutely angled, and skin sutures should be too tight. Skin flaps should be thick enough that there is no risk of necrosis.

7.3.5 Safety Principles for the Midlateral Approach to the Flexor Sheaths

- The palmar digital nerve is at risk if the skin incision and approach are too far in the volar direction. This approach is to be begun just dorsal to the end of the interphalangeal creases, where the palmar digital nerve is well protected.
- The volar digital artery goes with the digital nerve on its inner side. It may be also injured if the surgical approach moves too far in a volar direction.

7.3.6 Safety Principles for the Volar Approach to the Scaphoid

- The radial artery runs very close to the lateral border of this surgical wound and can be injured accidently at any time during the surgical dissection. It must be identified early in the procedure.

7.3.7 Safety Principles for the Dorsolateral Approach to the Scaphoid

- The superficial radial nerve is in danger during this surgical approach. Because it lies on the tendon of the extensor pollicis longus muscle, it is easy to injure as the tendon is mobilized.
- Injuring this nerve accidently may lead to an area of hypoesthesia on the dorsal aspect of the hand and a bothersome neuroma.
- Utmost care must be taken while operating on the hand and wrist since injury to the nerve can produce a great disability. The dominant hand must also be acknowledged.

7.3.8 Safety Principles for Arthroscopic Wrist Surgery

- Wrist arthroscopy has become an established investigative tool and is starting to be a useful therapeutic technique as well. All the extensor tendons, the radial artery, and dorsal sensory nerve branches are at risk during this surgical procedure, but fully understanding the periportal anatomy will make wrist arthroscopy a safer surgery. A good technique of establishing wrist arthroscopy portals is highlighted here.
- The 1-2, 6R, and 6U portals are the most risky, while the midcarpal, 3-4, 4-5, and distal radioulnar joint portals are comparatively safe. Even "safe" portals have occasional adjacent sensory nerve branches and tendon injuries.
- The primary radiocarpal portal, the 3-4, is created 1 cm distal to Lister's tubercle and just above the distal radius. The adjacent extensor pollicis longus angles radially, providing an ideal portal ulnar to the extensor pollicis longus and radial to the extensor digitorum communis tendons, between the scaphoid, lunate, and radius.
- The 6R portal is lateral to the extensor carpi ulnaris and distal to the ulnar head. The 6U portal is just medial to extensor carpi ulnaris.
- The 6U portal is made just palmar to the anterior margin of the extensor carpi ulnaris tendon and proximal to the medial prominence of the triquetrum. While an arthroscopic traction device restricts the forearm rotation, the 6U portal should not be made under traction with the hand fully pronated. Failure to implement this precaution can jeopardize the dorsal sensory branch of ulnar nerve.

- The 1-2 portal is made between the first and second extensor compartment tendons, and the 4-5 portal is at the interval of the fourth and fifth extensor compartment tendons.
- A volar radiocarpal portal is created at the radial volar wrist, at the level of the joint just lateral to the flexor carpi radialis tendon and medial to the radial artery, which is felt and marked well before the tourniquet is inflated.
- The midcarpal radial portal is made on a line along the lateral side of the third metacarpal, proximal to the capitates in the soft spot and about 1 cm distal to the 3-4 portal. The midcarpal ulnar portal is made on a line over the center of the fourth metacarpal, proximal to the capitate-hamate joint.
- The two main volar portals presently used are the volar radial portal and the volar ulnar portal, as described. The recently introduced volar central portal for wrist arthroscopy is centered on the lunate and used to view through the midcarpal and radiocarpal regions by a single incision. It starts in the distal wrist crease, which parallels the midcarpal joint, and extends 1.5 cm proximally up to the proximal wrist crease, which corresponds to the radiocarpal joint. The volar structures that are in danger are protected by retractors and also by tendons, to minimize the chance of injury. This portal may be useful in ligamentoplasties, arthroscopic arthrodesis, proximal row carpectomies, and other advanced procedures.

7.3.9 Safety Principles for the Drainage of Pus in the Hand

- The digital nerves may be injured if the skin incision is made too far proximally.
- The fibrous septa connecting the distal phalanx to the skin make this an ideal location for collection of pus. Take care to incise all the loculi so that sufficient drainage takes place.
- While incising and draining the web space infection, both the digital nerves and vessels of the web space are vulnerable.
- While incising the tendon sheath infection, the digital neurovascular bundle is protected if the skin incision is made just above the dorsal end of the proximal and distal interphalangeal creases.
- While draining the midpalmar space, bear in mind that the digital nerves to the little and ring fingers run just below the palmar aponeurosis and cross the line of the skin incision. The digital arteries run along with the digital nerves and also may be at risk. The digital arteries should be seen and protected well before the palmar aponeurosis is incised.
- While draining the thenar space infection, the digital nerves to the index finger may get injured because they are in line with the skin incision. Care should be taken when incising the palmar aponeurosis.
- The motor branch to the thenar muscles branches out from the deep surface of the median nerve as it leaves the carpal tunnel, but the location of its division varies considerably. This nerve winds around the distal end of the flexor retinaculum to supply the muscles. The surgeon must protect the branch at the proximal end of the incision.

- While attempting to incise the radial bursa in the thenar region in a midlateral approach to the thumb, if the incision is made too far in the volar direction, the radial neurovascular bundle may be injured unintentionally.
- The digital nerve to the lateral side of the little finger is at risk if the skin incision for draining the ulnar bursa on the finger is made too far in a volar direction. The distal vessels run along with the nerves.

7.4 Discussion

A standard arthroscopic examination can reveal defects in the wrist joint that are missed by other diagnostic modalities, including arthrograms and MRI. Over the past two decades, the use of wrist arthroscopy in both the diagnosis and management of challenges in the wrist has grown tremendously [10]. A learning curve can be defined as an improvement in performance over time or with increasing experience or training. It has been shown that both a disciplined practice of the technique (>25 wrist arthroscopies per year) and the number of years of experience (>5 years) reduce the complications considerably [3]. In the United States, arthroscopy should be considered when a patient's wrist pain has persisted despite nonoperative treatment with splinting and/or occupational therapy delivered by a certified hand therapist [12]. The mean incidence of neurologic injury after wrist arthroplasty is 4.6%; injury to the median nerve injury occurs at a rate of 16.5% [2]. The volar portal should be approached with great caution [12].

Understanding the patterns of iatrogenic neurovascular injuries associated with wrist and hand surgeries is vital for orthopaedic and hand surgeons [2]. The incidence of resurgery in the distal radius is higher for patients treated with plating than for patients managed with pins or external fixation. Dorsal plating has fewer neurologic injuries than volar plating. Open carpal tunnel release has fewer neurologic complications than endoscopic release [2, 13]. Arthrodesis for chronic wrist pain and disability is associated with a 10% to 25% incidence of postoperative carpal tunnel syndrome [2].

It is highly recommended that all health establishments implement an antibiotic stewardship program and safety protocols to prevent and manage surgical site infections [14–18] (see also Chap. 1).

References

1. Seigerman D, Lutsky K, Fletcher D et al (2019) Complications in the management of distal radius fractures: how do we avoid them? *Curr Rev Musculoskelet Med* 12(2):204–212
2. Verdecchian N, Johnson J, Baratz M, Orebaugh S (2018) Neurologic complications in common wrist and hand surgical procedures. *Orthop Rev (Pavia)* 10(1):7355
3. Leclercq C, Mathoulin C (2016) Members of EWAS. Complications of wrist arthroscopy: a multicenter study based on 10,107 arthroscopies. *J Wrist Surg* 5(4):320–326
4. Beredjiklian PK, Bozentka DJ, Leung YL, Monaghan BA (2004) Complications of wrist arthroscopy. *J Hand Surg Am* 29(3):406–411

5. Adams BD (2010) Complications of wrist arthroplasty. *Hand Clin* 26(2):213–220
6. Esplugus M, Lluch A, Garcia-Elias M, Llisà-Pérez M (2014) How to avoid ulnar nerve injury when setting the 6U wrist arthroscopy portal. *J Wrist Surg* 3(2):128–131
7. Mathews AL, Chung KC (2015) Management of complications of distal radius fractures. *Hand Clin* 31(2):205–215
8. Abrams RA, Petersen M, Botte MJ (1994) Arthroscopic portals of the wrist: an anatomic study. *J Hand Surg Am* 19(6):940–944
9. Hoppenfeld S, de Boer P, Buckley R (2022) *Surgical exposures in orthopaedics: the anatomic approach*, 6th edn. Wolters Kluwer, Philadelphia
10. Auerbach D, Poehling GG. Wrist arthroscopy techniques. Smith & Nephew Wrist Series Technique Guide. https://www.smith-nephew.com/global/assets/pdf/products/surgical/wrist_arthroscopy_tg.pdf.
11. Corella F, Ocampos M, Del Cerro M et al (2016) Volar central portal in wrist arthroscopy. *J Wrist Surg* 5(1):80–90
12. Michelotti BF, Chung KC (2017) Diagnostic wrist arthroscopy. *Hand Clin* 33(4):571–583
13. Navarro CM, Pettersson HJ, Enocson A (2015) Complications after distal radius fracture surgery: results from a Swedish nationwide registry study. *J Orthop Trauma* 29(2):e36–e42
14. World Health Organization. Antimicrobial stewardship programmes in health-care facilities in low- and middle-income countries: a WHO practical toolkit. Published 2019. https://www.who.int/publications/i/item/9789241515481
15. National Institute for Health and Care Excellence. Antimicrobial stewardship: systems and processes for effective antimicrobial medicine use. NICE guideline 15. Published August 18, 2015. https://www.nice.org.uk/guidance/ng15
16. National Institute for Health and Care Excellence. Surgical site infections: prevention and treatment. NICE guideline 125. Published 2019. https://www.nice.org.uk/guidance/ng125
17. Seligman KM, Katz D, Farber MK (2018) Preventing surgical site infection after cesarean delivery: the anesthesia professional's role. *APSF Newsletter* 33(1):25–27
18. World Alliance for Patient Safety. Safe surgery saves lives: the second global safety challenge. World Health Organization website. Published 2009. https://www.who.int/patientsafety/safesurgery/knowledge_base/SSSL_Brochure_finalJun08.pdf

Safe Spine Surgery

8

8.1 Introduction

The field of spine surgery has evolved appreciably over the past three decades, with many advances in instrumentation and technique. Spine surgery has many common operative procedures to treat radiculopathy, myelopathy, instability caused by degeneration or trauma, infection, and tumors. Surgical techniques include decompression of neural elements and stabilization through an anterior, posterior, or combined approach. The surgical complication rate is reported as 25% after cervical, 17% after thoracic, and 32% after lumbar spine procedures [1]. Deep venous thrombosis and pulmonary embolism are among the possible complications of spinal surgery [1–4].

Major complications have been noted even after minimally invasive spine surgeries and vertebral augmentation procedures for osteoporotic vertebral compressive fractures, including cement leaks in vertebroplasty [5] and other grievous complications, ranging from 48% to 74% after spine surgeries [6]. Wrong-site surgery has also been reported all over the world [6].

Spinal trauma often leads to a complex interaction of injuries in the musculoskeletal and nervous systems. The blend of unique biomechanical and neurologic factors provides an exceptional challenge to the surgeon managing the spinally injured patient. Complications after spine fracture surgery have been extensively reported [3, 7].

Emergency decompression for acute cervical spinal cord injury remains an acceptable surgical decision today and has to be performed safely. However, optimal timing of operation is a result of a complex range of variables related to the health establishment, the patient, and the surgical team. In polytrauma situations, life-threatening injuries need to be treated immediately, followed by the salvage of threatened limb. If decompression of spinal cord is advocated. earliest possible intervention may be desirable [8, 9].

S. V. Babu, *Safe Orthopaedic Surgery*,
https://doi.org/10.1007/978-981-16-2846-7_8

8.2 Principles of Safe Spine Surgery [1–4, 7, 10–17]

The surgeon must possess a detailed anatomic understanding in spine surgical approaches and precise skills for safe surgery (Fig. 8.1). Marking the surgical site with precise identification of the level of vertebrae and accurate instrumentation technique are all needed for patient safety in spine surgery.

Anaesthesia and proper patient positioning also play a vital role in the safety of the patient. A supportive anaesthetist colleague who is able to produce a controlled hypotension to reduce blood loss and effectively manage other physiological factors will yield good results. Several general complications can happen in spinal surgery following anaesthesia and positioning, including wound infection and discitis, cervical traction, dural tear, and cerebrospinal fluid leak. These factors must be acknowledged with great precaution.

8.2.1 Safety Principles for Preventing General Complications in Spine Surgery

- The reported incidence of postoperative respiratory compromise varies from 0% to 14%. Avoiding prolonged prone position and manual inline axial stabilization with fiberoptic nasal or oral endoscopy will reduce the risk of spinal cord injury during tracheal intubation. Patients with cervical instabilities must be given paramount care in providing general anaesthesia.
- Maintaining adequate blood pressure is vital for neural perfusion. Same-time controlled hypotension reduces blood loss and facilitates spine surgical exposure.
- Proper positioning of the patient is key to permitting full access in the surgical field and is necessary to avoid pressure that causes iatrogenic injuries. Areas to

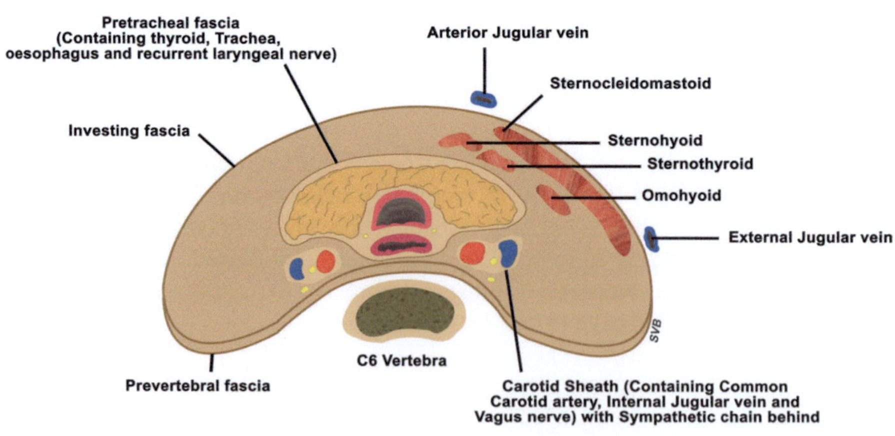

Fig. 8.1 The sixth cervical vertebra and its neurovascular relations

be safeguarded include the face, iliac crests, lower ribs, patella ,and anterior region of the ankle joints.

- Excessive traction with the tape or extension of shoulders inferior to the coracoid process is to be avoided to prevent compression of the brachial plexus. The technique of hanging the arm over the edge of the surgical table can injure the radial nerve and should be avoided. Injury to the common peroneal nerve can occur if the legs are placed in abduction and external rotation, which will cause pressure over the fibular head. Adequate padding below the pressure points will prevent skin and peripheral nerve injuries, especially in prolonged prone positioning.
- Sufficient head and neck control is compulsory to prevent damage to the spinal cord, such as skeletal traction via a halo ring or Mayfield tongs. Being in the prone position for extended periods can increase intraocular pressure, which will lead to ischemia, decreased perfusion pressure, and decreased blood supply to the retina, which can result in ischemic optic neuropathy, blindness, and occipital stroke. Pressure over the eyeballs is to be avoided by use of a Mayfield headrest or Gardner-Wells tongs. The upper limbs are kept by the side, and the shoulders are usually pulled distally and strapped to the surgical table to facilitate lateral radiography.
- Local complications due to cervical traction pins include tract infection, dura penetration leading to leakage of cerebrospinal fluid, brain abscess and meningitis, dissemination of fractures in presence of minimal skull fractures, loss of fixation, complications of hanging weights, arterial injuries, overdistraction and related disc protrusion, missing the distraction type of cervical injuries, and pin malpositioning. Injury to the temporal artery can be caused by the traction pins due to direct laceration or pin site invasion. The perfect pin site is at the thickest skull bone, located above the external auditory meatus bilaterally. The area at the anterosuperior segment of the ear tragus is to be avoided.
- Overdistraction is dangerous in occipitocervical dislocations and odontoid fractures. Hyperextension is also to be avoided. Cranial nerve injury involving the abducens, glossopharyngeal, vagus, and hypoglossal nerves has also been documented after traction with an incidence of 0.07%
- The risk of durotomy during laminectomy is reported to be 0.3–13% and can be up to 18% with revision surgery. Risk factors include old age, thin dura as a result of chronic compression, ossification of the ligamentum flavum, synovial cysts, and scarring from previous surgeries. The ligamentum flavum and posterior longitudinal ligaments are useful barriers during decompression, and these soft tissues must be carefully dissected after the overlying bone is removed.

8.2.2 Safety Principles for Anterior Cervical Spine Surgery

8.2.2.1 Preventing Recurrent Laryngeal, Superior Laryngeal, and Hypoglossal Nerve Injuries

- Safe dissection is advised in both left- and right-sided approaches. Avoiding the lateral ligature of the inferior thyroid vessels will safeguard against recurrent laryngeal nerve injury.

- Use of sharp-toothed retractors is advised; placing them under the longus colli muscle belly and avoiding the tracheoesophageal groove will prevent vocal cord paralysis
- Endotracheal tube accounts for 11.2% of vocal cord paralysis. Too much inflation of the tube must be avoided since it will produce retraction pressure against the larynx in causing nerve injury
- Reaching the upper spine (C2–C4) requires much care in preventing superior laryngeal nerve and hypoglossal nerve injury since these nerves may resemble blood vessels.

8.2.2.2 Preventing Esophageal Injury

- As discussed above, the retractors must be carefully placed, and displacement anteromedially can compress the trachea and esophagus medially. This can be prevented by intermittent release of the retractors.
- Esophageal perforation has an incidence of 0.2–1.15%. To avoid this, blunt finger dissection is recommended for exposure below the superficial cervical fascia. Also, proud screw fixation must be avoided since the posterior esophageal mucosa is very delicate. Perforation of the esophagus is a nasty problem that can lead to various dangerous complications like mediastinitis, retropharyngeal abscess, pneumonia, and tracheoesophageal fistula. Immediate attention has to be given to perforation since it has a 50% mortality rate. Emergency repair or flap coverage must be performed in the same setting.

8.2.2.3 Preventing Vertebral and Carotid Artery Injuries

- Injury to vertebral artery has an incidence of 0.3–0.5%. Damage occurs most often during surgery anterior to the transverse foramen of C7 or during lateral compression maneuvers from C3 to C6. Meticulous identification of the longus colli and uncovertebral joints is crucial for midline dissections.
- Dissection must be precise and retractors must be placed as mentioned earlier, as displacement anterolaterally can damage the carotid artery. This can be prevented by intermittent release of the retractors.

8.2.2.4 Preventing Tracheal Injury

- Tracheal injury can be life-threatening as the defect may allow the esophagus to prolapse into the tracheal lumen, causing acute asphyxia. It must be repaired immediately with or without sternocleidomastoid muscle flap coverage.
- Tracheal injury can be also prevented by placing the retractors carefully, as displacement anteromedially can put pressure on the trachea medially.

8.2.2.5 Preventing Thoracic Duct and Cervical Sympathetic Chain Injury

- Thoracic duct injury can occur during left-sided neck dissection. The thoracic duct can be identified dorsal to the subclavian vein and should be protected. It may lead to chylorrhea and chylous fistula.

- The cervical sympathetic chain travels between the carotid sheath and longus colli. It must be carefully preserved in midcervical approaches. Any aggressive retraction in surgery lateral to the longus colli can cause injury.

8.2.2.6 Preventing Pharyngocutaneous Fistula

- Pharyngocutaneous fistula may result from the esophageal injuries during dissection, while using a bur tool for decompression, or during instrumentation of the anterior cervical spine.

8.2.2.7 Preventing Spinal Cord and Nerve Root Injuries

- These injuries are caused while the osteophyte is being removed with Kerrison ronguers or by drilling. Thorough hemostasis, adequate illumination and visualization, experience, and correct technique are important in avoiding this insult. Spinal cord injury can also occur while the bone graft is being inserted after discectomy. Ensuring suitable sizing and carefully shaping and tapping the graft in place with correct depth and height can prevent bone graft extrusion.
- Electrophysiologic monitoring using somatosensory and motor-evoked potentials of the spinal cord is useful for monitoring during surgery and is especially beneficial in high-risk patients who have preexisting cord contusion or severe stenosis. Preoperative baselines are to be obtained in patients for comparison.

8.2.2.8 Preventing Adjacent Segment Degeneration

- Adjacent segment degeneration develops after 15% of anterior cervical discetomy and fusion surgeries and 9% of all posterior surgeries. This complication is less likely to develop after fusionless surgery. Plating can speed up adjacent segment degeneration if it is placed within 8 mm of the adjacent cranial disc segment, which is to be avoided.

8.2.2.9 Preventing Pseudarthrosis

- The incidence of pseudarthrosis ranges widely, from 0% to 50%. Surgeons should avoid prescription of drugs like nonsteroidal anti-inflammatory drugs and phenytoin for at least 10 weeks before surgery and avoid placing bone substitutes like bone morphogenic protein in fusion surgery in sensitive areas, such as behind esophagus.

8.2.3 Safety Principles for Corpectomy

- The overall morbidity associated with corpectomy is 11–27%. Unlike discectomy, corpectomies carry a greater risk of graft migration, strut graft dislodgement, infection, insufficient deformity correction, failure of fixation, neurologic insult, and pseudarthrosis because of major destabilization of the anterior column of the spine.
- Late complications are graft fracture, collapse or subsidence, and nonunion. Most graft dislodgments occur shortly after surgery (within 24 h). Graft migra-

tion rates will increase appreciably with each additional fusion level, with a reported odds ratio of 1.65. Additional external immobilization with a halo vest can theoretically increase the rigidity of the construct and decrease the chance of cage dislodgment, especially in longer fusions.

- Graft displacement and subsidence are significant problems with anterior surgery that can be avoided by careful patient selection and surgical technique. Excellent preparation of the graft, obtaining parallel fusion beds, and placing the graft under load from the cortical bone are key steps to ensuring the maximum stability for fusion.

8.2.4 Safety Principles for Surgery for Ossified Posterior Longitudinal Ligament

- The reported complications after ossified posterior longitudinal ligament surgery are noteworthy—about 2–10% incidence of quadriplegia and 5–7% chance of C5 root injury. Added lateral decompression is needed as the ligament expands laterally at the intervertebral disc level. This surgery also carries the danger of injuring the vertebral artery if dissection is lateral to the uncinate process.

8.2.5 Safety Principles for Cervical Disc Arthroplasty/Replacement

- The general complications are comparable between fusion and disc replacement. Patients with osteoporosis must avoid disc arthroplasties, as good bone quality is needed for tight prosthesis fitting. Patients with facet degeneration and severe vertebral collapse should not undergo disc replacement.

8.2.6 Safety Principles for Posterior Cervical Spine Surgery

8.2.6.1 Preventing Spinal Cord and Nerve Root Injuries

- The incidence of spinal cord and nerve root injuries is 0.18% and increases with severe cervical kyphosis correction (2.6%). Late neurologic complications can be prevented in posterior corrective surgery for cervical kyphosis by prophylactic foraminotomies in the case of foraminal stenosis, kyphosis correction that does not exceed 9.7° per spinal segment, and avoidance of kyphosis correction at C4–C5, which is where the largest posterior shift of the spinal cord happens, which can lead to C5 palsy. This is a frequent setback but in most cases it resolves spontaneously. As in anterior surgery, monitoring the spinal cord is an excellent resource.

8.2.6.2 Preventing C5 Palsy

- A 3.4% incidence of early postoperative C5 nerve root deterioration has been reported. These injuries are usually motor dominant but may also have sensory and radicular pain. C5 dysfunction can occur immediately to 20 days later. Recovery usually occurs but may take weeks, months, or as long as 6 years. Traction injuries to the nerve root are the expected insult due to the posterior bulge of the decompressed cord. The C5 root is in danger because of its direct and short course as it comes out from the spinal cord. It is also at the apex of lordosis. Hence, the distance of cord shift and root traction is more. With a posterior drift, C5 root tethering can occur, and it may be stretched beyond its tolerance limit. The deltoid has a single innervation from the C5 nerve root, so any nerve disruption has a reflective effect on patient function. The prophylactic foraminotomy is to be considered in patients with preexisting deltoid weakness, intervertebral foraminal stenosis, ossified posterior longitudinal ligament, and laminectomy along with instrumentation.

8.2.6.3 Preventing Spring-Back Closure

- This complication been reported at the rate of 40%. It occurs only in cervical open door laminoplasty. Special suturing techniques and bone graft will prevent this.

8.2.6.4 Preventing Postlaminectomy Kyphosis

- The incidence of kyphosis deformity following multilevel laminectomy is about 20%. Older patients might have partially fused cervical spines, and they are more stable. Postoperative kyphosis is quiet common in younger patients, however. Laminectomy is to be avoided in younger patients without cervical lordosis. Posterior facet joints are not to be damaged intraoperatively. Fusion during the same surgery must be considered for these patients.

8.2.7 Safety Principles for Screw Fixation in Cervical Spine

- This highly technical procedure must be carefully done. Screw malposition occurs about in up to 4% pf cases in the atlas up to 7% in the axis. Transarticular C1–C2 screws or Magerl screws cause an additional risk of vertebral artery injury, neurologic injury, or insufficient bony purchase. Vertebral artery injury is one of the most hazardous complications of screw fixation and is usually due to incorrect cervical pedicle screw entry. The incidence of iatrogenic vertebral artery injury is 1.3–4% in Magerl fixation. Lateral deviation of screws usually leads to penetration of the foramen transversalis, causing vertebral artery injury. Current trends include the use of intraoperative CT and computer-assisted navigation systems to improve screw trajectory and thereby reduce screw perforation.

- Subaxial lateral mass screws carry a danger in causing nerve root injury (1.3%) and a lateral mass fracture. Direct nerve root injury during lateral mass screw insertion can be avoided with image intensifier usage. Insertion under sagittal angulations of less than 15° may cause impingement on the exiting nerve root by the protrusion of screw threads. In axial trajectories of more than 30° lateral to the midline, lateral mass fracture (1.6%) or screw cut-out (1.3%) may happen. However, neurologic harm is rare. Screws placed too medially also can injure the vertebral artery.

8.2.8 Safety Principles for Posterior Occipitocervical Instrumentation

- In occipitocervical instrumentation, accurate insertion of the occipital screws is vital in preventing complications. Any screws inserted above the superior nuchal line can damage the transverse sinus. Loosening of screws is reported in 4.2–7% of cases, and dural tears happen in up to 4.2% while drilling the occiput and during screw placement. This region of the scalp is also quite thin, and skin erosion due to prominent implants is also possible. Dural laceration can occur during drilling of the occiput using bur hole or while using wire recoil for wire-based fixation (25–28%). Dural laceration will cause cerebrospinal fluid leak, but insertion of screw in the drill hole is usually adequate to stop it. Late complications of occipitocerivcal fusion are pseudarthrosis (6%) and adjoining level of degeneration (7%).

8.2.9 Safety Principles for Minimally Invasive Cervical Spine Surgery

- The limited visualization offered by minimally invasive spine surgery can lead to more damaging complications. Manipulation in a tight neural foramen can result in nerve root injury. Direct spinal cord injury may also occur during dilation or decompression. Using an imaging system while inserting the blunt dilator is advocated to prevent it from entering the interlaminar space and to prevent nerve injury. Dural tears have been reported in 1.6–6.6% of minimally invasive decompression procedures, and conversion to open surgery is usually needed to repair the dura.

8.2.10 Safety Principles for Vertebral Augmentation in Osteoporotic Fractures

- In this unique procedure, patient selection and radiographic evaluation are the most important criteria. The procedure is performed with the patient in the prone position, and the vertebroplasty/kyphoplasty needle is placed in the vertebral body either through a transpedicular or parapedicular approach. Utmost care must be taken not to cross to the medial or inferior aspect of the pedicle, which can damage the thecal sac, spinal cord, or nerves [5].

8.2.11 Safety Principles for Pedicle Screw Fixation

- This procedure is technically challenging and associated with a high complication rate. Screw misplacement (6.5%) and screw breakage (12.4%) inevitably lead to loss of correction. Inadequate fixation and subsequent motion also produce significant morbidity in patients. To prevent screw breakage and subsequent loss of correction, anterior support is to be provided through either posterior or anterior lumbar interbody fusion (PLIF or ALIF) techniques in case of post-spondylolisthesis L5-S1 reduction.
- The other important complication in pedicle screw fixation is nerve root irritation from medial angulations of the screw with disruption of the medial cortex of the pedicle.
- The most favorable screw placement is classically along the medial aspect of the pedicle. The instrumentation will get purchase from its proximity to cortical bone but must not damage it; the tip of the pedicle screw must not breach the anterior cortex of the vertebral body. Complications will arise from medial or lateral intrusion of a screw or from its insulting the anterior cortex of the vertebral body. The same complications will arise from malpositioning of anterior cervical plates and screws, which may disrupt the adjacent disc space, foramen transversarium, spinal cord, or nerve roots. Graft material in either case may also herniate anteriorly or posteriorly and cause neurologic compromise.
- The ideal pedicle screw must have the greatest diameter and length without insulting the pedicle's cortical layer or that of the vertebral body and it must converge.

8.2.12 Safety Principles for Preventing Deep Venous Thrombosis and Pulmonary Embolism

- Low-molecular-weight heparin regimens reduce the frequency of deep venous thrombosis and pulmonary embolism in spinal surgery. Mechanical prophylaxis also reduces the incidence of these complications.

8.2.13 Safety Principles for Preventing Surgical Site Infection in Spine Surgery

- The incidence of SSI in spine surgery is 0.1–4.7%. *Staphylococcus aureus* is the most common organism involved. The risk may be due to patient factors like obesity, diabetes mellitus, immunosuppression, steroid usage, or extremes of age, or procedural factors like longer operating time, more bleeding, more tissue trauma, and more staff movements while operating.

- It is highly recommended that all health establishments implement an antibiotic stewardship program and safety protocols to prevent and manage surgical site infections [10, 13] (see also Chap. 1).
- Proper education is important with regard to surgery and the postoperative period. Antibiotic prophylaxis should be given starting 15–30 min before surgery, either cefuroxime 1.5 g or 2 g IV BD for 24 h postoperatively, or for 48 h postoperatively for implant surgery. Surgical site hair removal is undertaken just before surgery (using clippers not razors) and the skin is prepped with chlorhexidine skin solution. Iodophor-impregnated drape should be used, which promotes less tissue injury and less diathermy usage.
- The anaesthesiologist's role is also a key factor in preventing surgical site infection, and the following protocols with phase of care will help in producing good results: mitigating risk factors, glycemic control, maintaining normothermia, antibiotic prophylaxis, and patient education [6].
- The duration of surgery is related to bacterial load. Operations longer than 3 h increase the chance of infection; more than 10^5 organisms can be found in surgical wounds after 5.7 h. A very high-quality surgical technique is fundamental for reducing infection. This includes careful dissection within avascular planes and potential dead spaces.

8.3 Discussion

Complications in spine surgery can produce personal and economic disruption that affects the quality of life and future freedom of patients. The North American Spine Society (NASS) had established a sign, mark, and x-ray (SMax) program for identification of exact patient and operation level [18]. This program has three key factors for patient safety in spine surgery:

- Patient identification and confirmation of medical records, including imaging studies and informed consents
- Surgical site markings
- Verification of the spine pathology level during operation using radiography

When executed watchfully and by the book, cervical spine surgery can be successful and have a low rate of untoward incidences. The surgeon's alertness must extend from induction of the anaesthesia and patient positioning to meticulous dissection and instrumentation techniques—that is, the entire procedure. In anterior surgery, prolonged and forceful retractions is to be avoided to preventi injury to the esophagus, recurrent laryngeal nerve, and carotid arteries. Further protection of corpectomies with plating combined with posterior spinal fusion and instrumentation will reduce the incidences of graft dislodgments. Careful selection of patients for corpectomy is the key factor since graft collapse and subsidence commonly occurs with osteopenic bone. In posterior surgery, prophylactic foraminotomy will reduce the risk of C5 nerve root palsy. Spinal cord monitoring should occur in all cases of cervical spine surgery. A very cautious analysis of the bony and vascular anatomy is to be done preoperatively, especially when internal fixation is planned. Preservation of posterior muscle and their attachments is vital for prevention of postoperative neck pain and delayed kyphosis.

Most complications are avoidable with sufficient preparation. Applying principles of antisepsis will prevent surgical site infection. Complications of spine surgery can sometimes be difficult to diagnose, and it is also frequently difficult to identify the reasons of recurrent symptoms on clinical grounds alone. Radiography is the benchmark follow-up imaging method [3, 6].

References

1. Proietti L, Scaramuzzo L, Schiro GR et al (2013) Complications in lumbar spine surgery: a retrospective analysis. *Indian J Orthop* 47(4):340–345
2. Jutte PC, Castelein RM (2002) Complications of pedicle screws in lumbar and lumbosacral fusions in 105 consecutive primary operations. *Eur Spine J* 11(6):594–598
3. Young PM, Berquist TH, Bancroft LW, Peterson JJ (2007) Complications of spinal instrumentation. *Radiographics* 27(3):775–789
4. Chahoud J, Kanafani Z, Kanj SS (2014) Surgical site infections following spine surgery: eliminating the controversies in the diagnosis. *Front Med (Lausanne)* 1:7
5. Barrocas AM, Eskey CJ, Hirsch JA (2007) Vertebral augmentation in osteoporotic fractures. *Injury* 38(suppl 3):588–596
6. Lee S-H, Kim J-S, Jeong Y-C et al (2013) Patient safety in spine surgery: regarding the wrong-site surgery. *Asian Spine J* 7(1):62–71
7. Gautschi OP, Schatlo B, Schaller K, Tessitore E (2011) Clinically relevant complications related to pedicle screw placement in thoracolumbar surgery and their management: a literature review of 35,630 pedicle screws. *Neurosurg Focus* 31(4):E8
8. Licina P, Nowitzke AM (2005) Approach and considerations regarding the patient with spinal injury. *Injury* 36(suppl 2):B2–B12
9. Fehlings MG, Perrin RG (2005) The role and time of early decompression for cervical spinal cord injury: update with a review of recent clinical evidence. *Injury* 36(suppl 2):B13–B26
10. World Alliance for Patient Safety. Safe surgery saves lives: the second global safety challenge. World Health Organization website. Published 2009. https://www.who.int/patientsafety/safesurgery/knowledge_base/SSSL_Brochure_finalJun08.pdf
11. Nasser R, Yadla S, Maltenfort MG et al (2010) Complications in spine surgery. *J Neurosurg Spine* 13(2):144–157
12. He B, Yan L, Xu Z et al (2014) Treatment strategies for the surgical complications of thoracic spinal stenosis: a retrospective analysis of two hundred and eighty three cases. *Int Orthop* 38(1).117–122
13. National Institute for Health and Care Excellence. Antimicrobial stewardship: systems and processes for effective antimicrobial medicine use. NICE guideline 15. Published August 18, 2015. https://www.nice.org.uk/guidance/ng15
14. Reis RC, de Oliviera MF, Rotta JM, Botelho RV (2015) Risk of complications in spine surgery: a prospective study. *Open Orthop J* 9:20–25

15. Cheung JPY, Luk KD-K (2016) Complications of anterior and posterior cervical spine surgery. *Asian Spine J* 10(2):385–400
16. National Centre for Disease Control. National treatment guidelines for antimicrobial use in infectious diseases. Directorate General of Health Services, Ministry of Health and Family Welfare, Government of India. Published 2016. https://ncdc.gov.in/WriteReadData/l892s/File622.pdf
17. Indian Council of Medical Research, Department of Health Research. Treatment guidelines for antimicrobial use in common syndromes. Published 2017. https://iamrsn.icmr.org.in/images/pdf/STG270217.pdf.
18. North American Spine Society. Prevention of wrong-site surgery: sign, mark, and X-ray (SMaX). Burr Ridge, IL; 2001. http://www.spine.org/Pages/PracticePolicy/ClinicalCare/SMAX/Default.aspx.

Safe Hip Surgery

9

9.1 Introduction

Surgical management is indicated for most hip diseases and fractures, be it a simple arthrotomy or a total revision hip replacement surgery. Hip fractures are common; the estimated worldwide incidence is more than 1.6 million annually [1]. The patients tend to be older and female and to have multiple comorbidities.

Basic principles of safe hip surgery include a complete knowledge of anatomy of the region and its variability, correct patient positioning, expert surgical skills for making adequate incisions and safe dissections that minimize bleeding and produce no damage to the vital structures [2].

Despite many advancements in surgical and anesthetic techniques, morbidity and mortality after hip surgery is significant, with both surgical and nonsurgical complications [3]. It has been reported that the complication rate is as high as 75% in hip surgeries. But formulating a system for, safe operations with early mobilization will reduce the number of complications and mortality [3, 4].

9.2 Applied Anatomy of the Hip Region (Fig. 9.1) [5]

9.2.1 Bony Landmarks

The anterosuperior iliac spine (ASIS), posterosuperior iliac spine (PSIS), greater trochanter, pubic tubercle, and pubic symphysis are key points in creating incisions for surgical approaches to the hip joint. These landmarks are to be protected and well padded.

S. V. Babu, *Safe Orthopaedic Surgery*,
https://doi.org/10.1007/978-981-16-2846-7_9

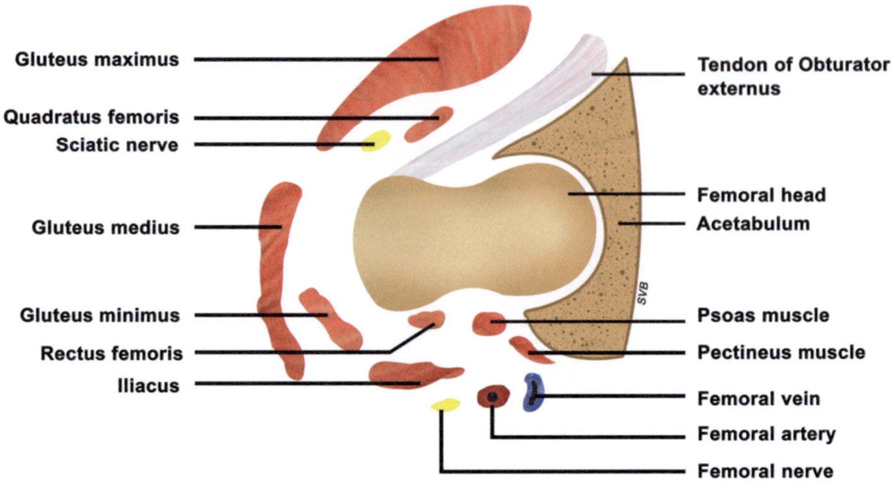

Fig. 9.1 The hip and its relations

9.2.2 Muscles

The gluteus medius and minimus should be taken much care since they are the prime hip stabilizers in the swing phase of the gait cycle. The iliopsoas tendon inserts posteromedially into the lesser trochanter. The piriformis is of great surgical importance in studying the neurovascular anatomy of the hip region. The superior gluteal vessels and nerve pass below this muscle.

9.2.3 Vessels

Although the incidence of major vascular injury during hip surgery is about 0.2–0.3%, such an injury can challenge the survival of the limb and the patient. The superior gluteal artery is in danger where it branches out at the upper border of piriformis. This danger spot is three fingerbreadths in front of the PSIS. The deep branch is also in danger as it traverses with the corresponding nerve about 4–6 cm superior to the acetabular rim. The lateral femoral circumflex artery, a branch of the profunda femoris artery, may get injured and requires ligation during the Smith-Petersen approach.

9.2.4 Nerves

The nerves of significance in hip surgeries are the lateral femoral cutaneous nerves, the femoral nerve, the superior and inferior gluteal nerves, the sciatic nerve, and the obturator nerve. The lateral femoral cutaneous nerve is the most disrupted during anterior approaches. The sciatic nerve has an important posterior relation to the hip.

The incidence of sciatic nerve injury associated with posterior approaches to the hip is estimated at 0.07–0.1%. The varied anatomy of the sciatic nerve in relationship to the piriformis should be well known to the surgeon. The nerve should be identified and safeguarded. The superior gluteal nerve has a high risk for injury, particularly in gluteus-splitting approaches. The safe area when splitting the abductors (gluteus medius) is 5 cm from the tip of the greater trochanter. The pathway of the superior gluteal nerve is as close as 3 cm from the tip of the greater trochanter.

9.2.5 Joint Capsule and Ligament

The hip capsule is the strong fibrous tissue that extends to the intertrochanteric line anteriorly; however, on the posterior surface, it is deficient. The capsule is strengthened anteriorly by the iliofemoral ligament of Bigelow, inferiorly by the pubofemoral condensation, and posteriorly by a thin ischiofemoral ligament. The ligamentum fovea runs from the fovea of the femoral head to the acetabular fovea.

9.3 Principles of Safe Hip Surgery [5]

9.3.1 Safety Principles for the Anterior Approach

- With the patient in the supine position, the skin incision is created starting at the middle of the iliac crest and moved anteriorly to the ASIS. From that point, the incision is done distally and just laterally for 8–10 cm. The space between the tensor fasciae latae and the sartorius is found by blunt dissection approximately 5–7.5 cm below the ASIS. The lateral femoral cutaneous nerve, which goes through the deep fascia close to the intramuscular interval, is noted and protected.
- The sartorius muscle is retracted above and medially, and then the tensor fasciae latae is retracted below and laterally. The ascending branch of the lateral circumflex femoral artery crosses here; it must be noted and protected. The deep dissection is done on the space between the rectus femoris muscle (supplied by the femoral nerve) and the gluteus medius muscle (supplied by the superior gluteal nerve). The rectus femoris is dissected from its origins and retracted medially while the gluteus medius is retracted laterally. The capsule of the hip joint is now visible.

9.3.2 Safety Principles for the Anterolateral Approach

- With the patient in the supine position, the skin incision begins at a point 2–3 cm posterior to the ASIS and is directed toward the mid-segment of the greater trochanter. It then runs 10–15 cm along the axis of the femur. Next, the fascia lata is incised and the space between the tensor fasciae latae and gluteus medius identified. It is bluntly divided between the ASIS and greater trochanter to

prevent injury to the inferior branch of the superior gluteal nerve, which supplies the tensor fascia latae.
- The gluteus medius and minimus are pulled proximally and laterally to expose the joint capsule. The ascending branch of the lateral circumflex femoral artery that goes deep to the tensor fasciae latae and gluteus medius needs to be safeguarded.

9.3.3 Safety Principles for the Lateral Approaches

9.3.3.1 Safety Principles for the Hardinge's Approach

- With the patient in the supine position, a clean lateral skin incision centered over the greater trochanter at exactly the center. After fascial dissection, the gluteus medius is seen and incised obliquely over the greater tochanter, leaving the posterior half with the trochanter. It is key to note that the abductor division should never be more than 5 cm above the tip of greater trochanter to prevent injury to the superior gluteal vessels and nerve. Then the gluteus minimus muscle is divided and pulled well proximally to allow visualization of the joint capsule.

9.3.3.2 Safety Principles for the Transtrochaneric Approach

- With the patient in the supine position, the gluteus medius and vastus lateralis at the greater trochanter are osteomized so that the muscles and a portion of bone are moved en bloc. There are lot of modifications of this technique available.

9.3.4 Safety Principles for the Posterior Approach

- The true lateral position is used for this approach. This commonly used technique for total hip replacement protects the abductor mechanism. The skin incision starts 10 cm from the PSIS and runs laterally and distally to the greater trochanter. It is moved distally 15 cm along the femoral shaft. After the fascia lata and gluteal fascial are divided in line with the skin incision, the gluteus maximus is dissected bluntly to ensure that the branches of the superior gluteal vessels and nerves in the proximal part of the muscle and those of the inferior gluteal vessels and nerve in the distal half of the muscle are safeguarded. The sciatic nerve is then visualized and protected. Also, the short external rotators are bluntly dissected and detached near their femoral insertion. The muscles are retracted medially to protect the sciatic nerve, and then the capsule is exposed.
- A well-repaired capsule after surgery is key to preventing dislocation.

9.3.5 Safety Principles for the Medial Approach

- With the patient in the supine position, the following maneuver is performed. The hip joint is flexed, abducted, and externally rotated to make the lesser trochanter and medial hip joint capsule closer to the skin surface. A 3-cm-long skin incision is made distal to the public tubercle in line with the adductor longus. The plane of dissection is between the adductor longus and gracilis by blunt dissection to make the superficial muscle interval. Deep dissection is conducted in the space between the adductor brevis and adductor magnus muscle. The adductor longus and brevis anterior muscles, along with the gracilis and adductor magnus, should be retracted. The posterior branch of the obturator nerve is viewed along the body of the adductor magnus. The anterior branch of the obturator nerve lying on the anterior surface of the adductor brevis is identified. Then the lesser trochanter is isolated at the base of the wound by blunt dissection, and the iliopsoas tendon is mobilized. This technique exposes the medial hip joint capsule well.

9.3.6 Safety Principles for Minimally Invasive Two-Incision Hip Surgery

- A 5-cm anterior skin incision is made over the femoral neck and is used to reach the acetabulum. A 3-cm posterior incision is made in line with the femoral canal and is used for femoral preparation.

9.4 Discussion

Hip operations are common surgeries in orthopaedics. There are array of surgical approaches to the hip, and no single approach is appropriate for all hip procedures. The surgeon must be conversant with the range of approaches.

The complication rate after any orthopaedic surgery is 12.7% in a well-established orthopaedic center [4]. Complications after hip fracture surgery depend on the fracture type and whether it is extracapsular or intracapsular. The main challenges in intracapsular fractures are mainly biological: vascularization of the femoral head and lack of periosteum (a major contributor to fracture healing) in the femoral neck. In extracapsular fractures, in contrast, the challenge is mechanical and relates to load bearing.

It has been established that knowledge of clinical anatomy of the operating region combined with specialist skills yield superior results, reducing reduce operating time significantly and preventing medical complications [2, 4, 6–8]. It has also been shown, however, that supervised residents in medical educational establishments carry out surgery to safety levels comparable to those of experienced orthopaedic surgeons [4].

It is estimated annual incidence of hip fractures is more than 600,000, with high mortality [1]. The introduction of integrated pathways for the management of hip fractures in Sweden and the United Kingdom has shown significant reductions in mortality [9, 10]. Preventing and managing medical complications are the key factors in reducing morbidity and mortality following hip surgeries. This can be accomplished by developing orthogeriatric units in which orthopaedic surgeons and their medical and intensivist colleagues use a systems-based protocol [2, 3, 11–13]. It is highly recommended that all health establishments implement an antibiotic stewardship program and safety protocols to prevent and manage surgical site infections [14–18] (see also Chap. 1).

References

1. Johnell O, Kanis JA (2006) An estimate of the worldwide prevalence and disability associated with osteoporotic fractures. *Osteoporos Int* 17(12):1726–1733
2. Guimarães Barros AA, Cardoso Mendes CH et al (2017) Efficacy evaluation of a protocol for safe hip surgery (total hip arthroplasty). *Rev Bras Ortop* 52(suppl 1):29–33
3. George Institute for Global Health. Management of hip fractures in older people in India. George Institute website. https://www.georgeinstitute.org/projects/management-of-hip-fractures-in-older-people-in-india
4. Panesar SS, Carson-Stevens A, Salvilla SA et al (2013) Patient safety in orthopedic surgery: prioritizing key areas of iatrogenic harm through an analysis of 48,095 incidents reported to a national database of errors. Drug Healthc Patient Saf 5:57–65
5. Onyemaechi N, Anyanwu E, Obikili E, Ekezie J (2014) Anatomical basis for surgical approaches to the hip. *Ann Med Health Sci Res* 4(4):487–494
6. Miller GE (1990) The assessment of clinical skills/competence/performance. *Acad Med* 65(9 suppl):S63–S67
7. Fehring TK, Mason JB (2005) Catastrophic complications of minimally invasive hip surgery. *J Bone Joint Surg Am* 87(4):711–714
8. Carpintero P, Caeiro JR, Carpintero R et al (2014) (2014) Complications of hip fractures: a review. *World J Orthop* 5(4):402–411
9. Meyer AC, Hedström M, Modig K (2020) The Swedish Hip Fracture Register and National Patient Register were valuable for research on hip fractures: comparison of two registers. *J Clin Epidemiol* 125:91–99
10. National Institute for Health and Care Excellence. Hip fracture: management. NICE clinical guideline 124. Published June 22, 2011. https://www.nice.org.uk/guidance/cg124
11. Theelen L, Bischoff C, Grimm B, Heyligers IC (2018) Current practice of orthopaedic surgical skills training raises performance of supervised residents in total knee arthroplasty to levels equal to those of orthopaedic surgeons. *Perspect Med Educ* 7(2):126–132
12. Willhuber GC, Stagnaro J, Petracchi M et al (2018) Short-term complication rate following orthopedic surgery in a tertiary care center in Argentina. *SICOT J* 4:26
13. Flikweert ER, Wendt KW, Diercks RL et al (2018) Complications after hip fracture surgery: are they preventable? *Eur J Trauma Emerg Surg* 44(4):573–580
14. World Health Organization. Antimicrobial stewardship programmes in health-care facilities in low- and middle-income countries: a WHO practical toolkit. Published 2019. https://www.who.int/publications/i/item/9789241515481
15. National Institute for Health and Care Excellence. Antimicrobial stewardship: systems and processes for effective antimicrobial medicine use. NICE guideline 15. Published August 18, 2015. https://www.nice.org.uk/guidance/ng15
16. National Institute for Health and Care Excellence. Surgical site infections: prevention and treatment. NICE guideline 125. Published 2019. https://www.nice.org.uk/guidance/ng125
17. Seligman KM, Katz D, Farber MK (2018) Preventing surgical site infection after cesarean delivery: the anesthesia professional's role. *APSF Newsletter* 33(1):25–27
18. World Alliance for Patient Safety. Safe surgery saves lives: the second global safety challenge. World Health Organization website. Published 2009. https://www.who.int/patientsafety/safesurgery/knowledge_base/SSSL_Brochure_finalJun08.pdf

Safe Femur Surgery 10

10.1 Introduction

In today's high-speed, highly mechanized world, it has become nearly impossible to escape accidents and injuries, even in children. Fractures of the femur are one such mishap. Surgery has been well established for the treatment of femur fractures in both adults and children. The aim of femur fracture management is to re-establish lower limb length and anatomic articular surface alignment and rotation, as well as to establish adequate fixation for early mobilization of the associated joint with minimal complications [1]. Femoral injuries must be treated with the utmost care so that the full functional outcome of the total lower limb is realized [2].

Despite improvement in implants, instrumentation, and techniques [3–5], considerable surgical complications can occur with femur surgery [2, 6–14]. A lot of these complications are related to technical errors [15, 16]. In fact, it has been well established that the surgeon's experience plays a more vital role than any specific implant used for treatment [17]. Improving patient safety is a main concern today, since surgical complications can be catastrophic for patients, surgeons, and institutions [11, 18].

Early operative treatment for peritrochanteric fractures (injuries in the intertrochanteric and subtrochanteric region) will reduce both mortality and morbidity. It also offers the best chance of early independency and reduces the challenges presented by extended bed rest [5, 19]. These fractures pose a major health issue in the elderly. They can be repaired with extramedullary devices, intramedullary nailing, or arthroplasty [16]. Technical difficulties arise for many reasons in all these procedures, but with fine instrumentation, good experience, and attention to each surgical step, these problems can be minimized [14].

In total hip replacement, the most frequently injured vessels are the external iliac artery and the common femoral artery. Arthroplasty and surgery of fractures of hip and femur are associated with both penetrating and nonpenetrating iatrogenic femoral arterial trauma. While uncommon, these complications have grave consequences

S. V. Babu, *Safe Orthopaedic Surgery*,
https://doi.org/10.1007/978-981-16-2846-7_10

on limb survival and function. Mechanisms of injury include drill bit overpenetration, sharp bone spikes, screw protruding beyond the medial border of the femur, distal locking screw in the proximal femoral nail, improperly positioned retractors, and excessive traction on the atherosclerotic vessel. Along with traction, forceful medial retraction anterior to the hip joint, hyperextension, and various maneuvers for dislocating the hip are causes of nonpenetrating vascular trauma in hip and femur surgeries. Vascular injury can occur due to inappropriate retractor positioning at the acetabulum or proximal femur during primary or revision arthroplasty of the hip.

Complex fractures of the proximal femur are mostly associated with femoral arterial injury. These injuries are demonstrated immediately or may present later as pseudoaneurysm [10, 11, 20–25]. In this case, vascular repair must be the performed first, then open fracture fixation, to achieve good outcome [26]. Femoral artery and vein injury after cerclage wiring of the shaft femur in revision hip arthroplasty been also reported [21]. Even in children undergoing hip surgery, iatrogenic iliac vein injury that endangered a child's life has been reported [27].

Intramedullary nailing of diaphyseal and metaphyseal femur fractures is one of the most celebrated operations in orthopaedic trauma surgery. Locked intramedullary nailing is the treatment of choice for femoral shaft fractures, and familiarity with potential complications and their association with the fracture patterns is much needed for the surgeons [20]. Pudendal neuropathy is a common complication (9%) that associated with the longitudinal traction of the lower limbs during fracture surgery, especially during the interlocking nailing procedure of the femur [28]. Care has to be taken and forceful traction avoided. There are many factors contributing injury of the superior gluteal nerve while cephalomedullary nailing of femoral fractures [2].

Proximal femoral nail antirotation with closed reduction at the earliest opportunity is the prime choice for the treatment of femoral intertrochanteric fractures. Unfortunately, the complication rate associated with proximal femoral nail antirotation ranges between 6.5% and 35.5%. Complications and the risk of fixation failure can be reduced with attention to making a precise entry point, to sufficient reaming of proximal femur, to passing the nail carefully to avoid varus, and to verifying distraction at the fracture site when placing the lag screw in the inferior part of neck in anteroposterior imaging view and central in the lateral view [17, 29]. The less-invasive stabilization system (LISS) and, more recently, the reverse femoral LISS plate, have also been tried for some of these fractures, particularly in obese patients and in difficult situations in which intramedullary nailing is not possible [17, 29].

Early reamed intramedullary nailing of femoral fractures provides exceptional fracture healing, rapid patient recovery, and few complications related to the methodology [4, 30]. Intramedullary nailing is also an effective treatment for impending and pathologic fractures caused by metastatic cancer. Both staged and simultaneous bilateral nailing have shown to be safe approaches in these cases, but simultaneous nailing has a higher survival rates and fewer perioperative complications than staged nailing [31].

Iatrogenic femoral neck fractures can occur as a complication of femoral nailing. Using the awl instrument in the wrong direction forcefully or creating multiple entry points in the trochanteric region will weaken the femoral neck, and the neck of femur may fracture when the nail is hammered in [32].

A 2016 study reported that superior gluteal nerve injury had occurred in 28% of patients and myogenic damage of gluteus medius and gluteus minimus muscles in 20% of patients after antegrade femoral intramedullary nailing through piriform fossa entry [33].

Titanium elastic nail system (TENS) fixation is an effective load-sharing management of diaphyseal fractures of the femur in correctly chosen patients 6–16 years of age if the principles are well applied, including precise section of nail diameters and nail positioning [34–39]. In addition, some surgeons have treated femoral shaft fractures in younger children (3–12 years) successfully and with fewer complications with elastic nails than with conservative hip spica casting [40]. The precurved TENS nails facilitate flexible nailing procedures [36]. In pediatric patients 13 years and older with femur shaft fractures, rigid intramedullary nailing is to be considered after assessing the risk-benefit ratio in order to avoid avascular necrosis of the femoral head after nailing [4, 41]. Heavier children have a higher rate of complications. Patients younger than 13 years old and weighing less than 55 kg can be safely managed with an elastic stable nail system, but older and heavier children should be treated with rigid fixation systems to avoid complications [42].

Two minimally invasive implants are available for the distal femoral fractures—LISS and distal femoral nailing. They are both good, with similar outcomes, and they are also superior to condylar plates with regard to infections and axial malalignments [42, 43]. LISS for distal femoral fractures will lead to good bone healing when performed with precise surgical technique and with care taken to restore axial alignment [44]. LISS offers many benefits in treatment of complex distal femoral fractures, including less blood loss, low infection, early mobility. Bicortical screws give good fixation and are advised for osteoporotic fractures [45]. The meta-analysis evidence has shown that no implant system is superior to other in all circumstances for distal femoral fractures. In addition, retrograde distal femoral nailing and LISS plating have similar postoperative complications [1]. The longer distal femoral nail has more vascular risk while locking onto the hip [43]. The role of arthroscopy is limited and useful only in a few cases of reducing distal femur epiphyseal fractures [43].

Heterotopic ossification of the hip after reamed intramedullary femoral is an uncommon complication [46]. The extensive soft tissue handling during surgery can cause hip abductor ischemia, and delayed mobilization after surgery, hypercalcemia, and spinal cord injury are contributory factors for this ossification. If symptomatic, surgical management is indicated [46].

External fixation is indicated when a fracture femur is present with severe soft tissue injury, head injury, or polytrauma (as damage-control orthopaedics), or when the fracture is a pathologic in origin [47, 48]. External fixation is associated with many complications, mainly pin tract infection (72%) and secondary fractures after the implant removal (22%) [49].

About 8% of complications in fracture femur surgery are implant related [18]. Many modifications of implants and techniques had been made in recent years for reliable, safe, and effective management. A new cephalomedullary nail is designed to reduce the risk of implant failure in intertrochanteric hip fractures by allowing for insertion of two interdigitating screws [18].

10.2 Applied Surgical Anatomy of the Femur and Thigh

10.2.1 Muscles and Nerves of the Thigh

There are three major groups:

1. The adductors of the hip are innervated by the obturator nerve lies in the medial section of the thigh.
2. The extensors of the knee are innervated by the femoral nerve and occupies the anterior section of the thigh.
3. The flexors of the knee are supplied by the sciatic nerve and present in the posterior region of the thigh.

10.2.2 Arteries and Veins of the Thigh

The femoral artery is the artery that passes through the thigh (Fig. 10.1). The main branch, the profunda femoris artery, is the key blood supply of the thigh musculature. It passes behind the adductor longus muscle, where the femoral artery passes in front to it. Thus, the muscle is enveloped by these two arteries.

Four of the perforating branches of the profunda femoris artery pass behind and crosses the medial compartment of the thigh.

The average distances to the femur are 9.24 to 9.87 mm and 27.27 to 27.81 mm for deep femoral and superficial arteries, respectively. This means that the deep femoral arteries frequently are damaged during surgery.

The saphenous vein is the chief superficial vein of the thigh.

10.2.3 Angles of the Femur

The femur has a natural anterior bow. The angle between the femoral shaft and the femoral neck varies but is typically about 130°. The femoral neck is anteverted 15° on the femoral shaft.

The distal femur has a trapezoid shape and is narrower anteriorly. It functions with the tibia and patella as two joints in three compartments. The femoral condyles project in back of the diaphyseal axis, which ends at the condylar-trochlea junction. The lateral slope of the condyle tilts 10° inward and forward, and the medial slope tilts 25° forward and outward.

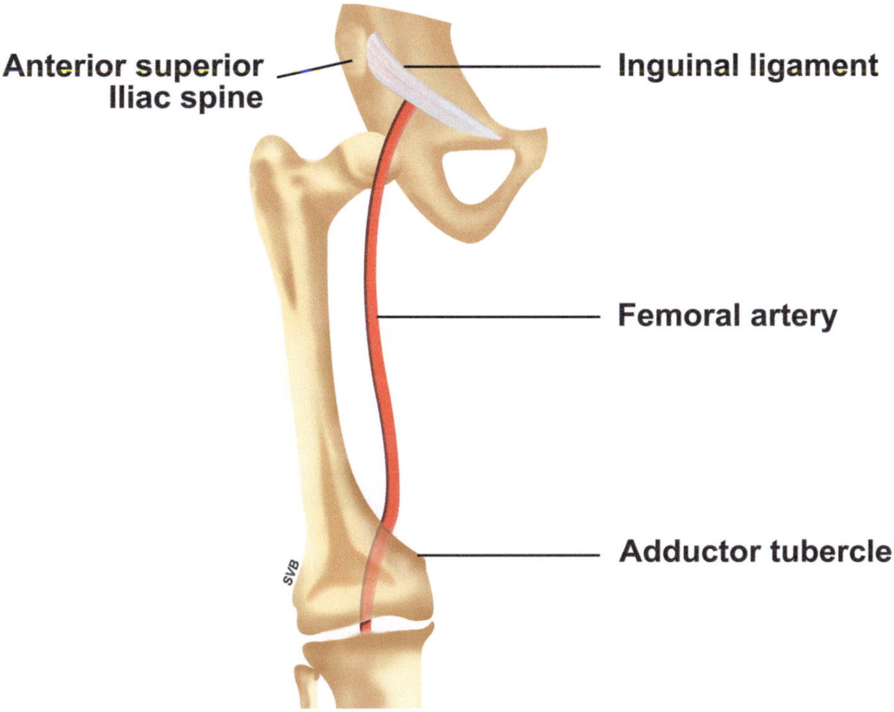

Fig. 10.1 The femur and its vascular relations

These angles are to be kept in mind when introducing pins or nails proximally and distally in the femur.

10.3 Principles of Safe Femur Surgery [16, 28, 35, 48, 50–58]

10.3.1 Safety Principles for the Lateral Approach to the Femur

- Many perforating branches of the profunda femoris artery go across the vastus lateralis muscle. They can be injured during this approach and should be safeguarded. These arterial branches can be seen more easily if the muscle is split gently with a blunt instrument rather than cut with a sharp instrument or knife.
- A novel method has been introduced recently for predicting safe zones in avoiding superior gluteal nerve injury, especially in the lateral approach to the hip. By measuring the trochanter to iliac crest distance preoperatively and using the respective standardized ratios, surgeons can precisely predict the nerve to trochanter distance, and the proximity of the superior gluteal nerve to the greater trochanter can be worked out with a more precise zone around the nerve to minimize the injury.

10.3.2 Safety Principles for the Anteromedial Approach to the Distal Two-Thirds of the Femur

- The medial superior genicular artery runs on the operative field just above the knee and goes around the lower end of the femur. Although it is small, it causes significant bleeding when injured.
- The lowest fibers of the vastus medialis muscle insert directly onto the medial border of the patella. This muscle is the main stabilizer of the patella in preventing lateral subluxation. It gets disrupted in this approach and has to be meticulously repaired.

10.3.3 Safety Principles for the Posterior Approach to the Femur

- The sciatic nerve runs down the back of the thigh in the posterior compartment. It lies medial to the biceps femoris muscle in the superior part of the incision.
- The nerve to the biceps femoris branches out from the sciatic nerve and enters the biceps from its medial side proximally in the thigh.

10.3.4 Safety Principles for the Posterolateral Approach to the Femur

- The perforating arteries branch out from the profunda femoris artery and go through the lateral intermuscular septum to supply the vastus lateralis muscle. They all have to be protected in the dissection process.
- The superior lateral geniculate artery and vein run on the lateral surface of the femur at the top of the femoral condyles.

10.3.5 Safety Principles for the Minimally Invasive Approach for LISS to the Distal Femur

- The superior genicular artery and veins are to be noted and ligated. These vessels may be numerous and are close to the periosteum. If they are injured in this approach, much bleeding will occur.
- The advised approaches for extra- and intra-articular distal femur fractures are different.
  - For extra-articular fractures, a skin incision is made from Gerdy's tubercle about 8 cm in the proximal direction. The iliotibial tract is split in the direction of the fibers. The interval between the lateral vastus and the periosteum is opened. Distally, the lateral vastus muscle is attached mainly on the femoral ridge. There are no muscle insertions on the lateral periosteum or bone. The internal fixator (LISS) can be inserted in the interval between the periosteum and the muscle.

  - For intra-articular fractures, an anterolateral arthrotomy is suggested. This procedure permits good control of the reduction and successive introduction of the LISS fixator, and can be used to introduce lag screws from medially.
- The superficial femoral artery comes very closely (median 21 mm) to the tip of the screw during LISS plate fixation of distal femur fractures. It can be closer to the line of drilling while using LISS plate holes number 6–10. Extra caution is needed while drilling in a lateral to medial direction in the high-risk plate zone.

10.3.6 Safety Principles for the Minimally Invasive Approach to the Proximal Femur for Intramedullary Nailing

- The correct entry is vital in intramedullary nailing of the femur.
- The nail introduction point for the proximal femoral nail should be at the modified medial trochanteric portal, which is just medial to the tip of the greater trochanter
- A nail entry point that is too far lateral is a common occurrence. This will establish a varus deformity at the fracture site if the nail used is rigid and the fracture is in the proximal third of the femur. Lateral entry can also produce an iatrogenic fracture of the medial femoral cortex during nail insertion.
- A nail entry point that is too far medial may also create an iatrogenic fracture of the femoral neck, usually a vertical basicervical fracture. Sometimes medial nail entry will also damage the blood supply to the femoral head, producing avascular necrosis.
- To prevent the loss of reduction of fracture fragments, they must be reduced and compressed by a medially directed force. Overreaming the proximal femur until the subtrochanteric region is reached also helps in protecting reduced fractures.
- The superior gluteal nerve runs posteriorly to anteriorly through the belly of the gluteus medius muscle 3–5 cm superior to the tip of the greater trochanter. If the femur is in adducted position, the nerve can be protected during insertion of a nail. The risk of injuring this nerve may be more with the patient in the standard supine position on the fracture table than with the patient in the lateral position, which affords greater hip flexion and adduction.
- Optimizing the tip–apex distance is decisive in preventing fixation crash when using an extramedullary sliding hip screw for fixing peritrochanteric fractures.

10.3.7 Safety Principles for the Minimally Invasive Approach to Retrograde Intramedullary Nailing of the Femur

- The infrapatellar branch of the saphenous nerve presents below the distal end of the incision. It is in danger only if the incision is carried out distally.
- The posterior cruciate ligament attaches to the lateral aspect of the medial femoral condyle. The insertion will get damaged by the intramedullary nail or the reamers used while creating the opening if the entry point is not aptly done.

10.3.8 Safety Principles for the Minimally Invasive Approach to TENS Nailing of the Femur

- The nail entry point should be at 2 cm from the physis of the femur. It should be above the flare of the medial and lateral condyles.
- The diameter of nail should be two-fifths of the internal diameter of the medullary canal (calculation: nail diameter = 0.4 × canal diameter).
- Ideally, the lateral nail must go to the level of the greater trochanter and the medial nail up to the femoral neck.
- The amount of prebending must be same for both the nails. It should be three times the inner diameter of the shaft.
- Care must be taken not to twist the nails more than 90° to avoid a corkscrew effect.
- When the nails both pass the fracture level, the traction has to released.

10.3.9 Safety Principles for Placing External Fixator Pins in the Femur

- The safe zone for anterior external fixator half-pin placement for the femur is an average of 20 cm in length only and can be narrow as 12 cm. The anterior pins must begin 6 cm below the lesser trochanter, with consideration of the nerves, and 7.5 cm above the superior pole of patella to avoid inadvertent knee joint penetration.
- Most arteries branching off the femoral artery cross posterior to the femur, supplying the vastus muscles as perforators. Although they can be injured during drilling or penetrated by the pins, their posterior location makes them less likely to be injured than nerves are.
- The entire lateral femur is safe for half-pin placement, distally beyond the synovial reflection of the suprapatellar pouch.
- Introduction of anterior external fixator pins into the distal femur must start at least 5 cm above the medial epicondyle or 5.5 cm above the lateral epicondyle to prevent entering the knee joint.
- The distal femoral traction pin should be inserted in a medial to lateral direction about 0.7 cm proximal to the adductor tubercle to avoid knee penetration.

10.3.10 Safety Principles for Reducing the Risk of Pudendal Nerve Palsy by Using a Fracture Table

- Application of adequate preoperative skeletal traction is required to avoid limb shortening.
- Complete muscular relaxation is indicated during surgery.
- Traction should be used only for trial reduction, guide wire passage, intramedullary nail passage, and placement of interlocking screws.
- Release the traction once the interlocking screws are placed.

- Fracture should be opened in case of difficulty.
- The final diameter of the perineal post should be 6.8–9 cm.

10.4 Discussion

The basic principles of intramedullary nailing should be well understood as a starting point for avoiding complications with this technique. Reported complications due to technical errors with intramedullary femoral nailing include malalignment, cut-out, infection, false drilling, wrong lag screw length and drill bit breakage during the interlocking procedure, external or internal malrotation (>20°) of the femoral diaphysis, elongation of the femur (2 cm), impaired bone healing, periprosthetic fracture distal to the tip of the nail, fracture collapse, implant failure, lag screw intrapelvic migration, neurovascular injury, secondary varus deviation, complications after implant removal, trochanteric pain and refracture [16, 59]. The frequent usage of bone awl and placing the nail entry too far medially can cause iatrogenic fracture of the femoral neck [60–63]. Establishing a proper entry point is the key factor in this surgery. The piriformis fossa is the best starting point from a mechanical aspect because it corresponds with the femoral canal; however, this increases the chance of damage to the medial circumflex artery, a concern especially in younger patients. The present generation of nails has a trochanteric portal that avoids injuring the vessels, however. Still, if the starting point of these nails is too lateral, it will force the hip into varus, leading to mechanical troubles and possibly inducing a blowout fracture of the medial cortex of the proximal femur [64].

The least strained and most anatomic point for safe nail insertion is in the line of the medullary canal of the femur, which can be located proximally on trochanteric area by calculating the trochanteric shaft angle (TSA) [65]. There can be individual variability in proximal femur anatomy, which can be related with the TSA to select the entry site for safe nail insertion. The nail entry precisely correlates with the proximal femoral anatomy, the type of nail (uniplanar or biplanar), anatomy of the greater trochanter, the TSA, the medullary canal, and the diameter of the nail. If the TSA is in between 0° and 6°, the point of entry should be at the center of the trochanteric region; if it is 6–12°, the entry should be at medial surface of the trochanter; for a TSA of 12–17°, the entry has to be even more medial to the greater trochanter, which may challenge the medial vascularity, and the biplanar nail has to used in this case [65].

The radius of curvature of femoral intramedullary nails does not match the average radius of curvature of the human femur; the nails are straighter than the anatomic curvature of the femur. This mismatch is not a challenge when the starting point is correct and when proper reduction and surgical technique are used in non-pathologic bone. However, anterior cortical injury does occur during nail fixation in some patients. Improper nail entry point and other technical errors contribute to the occurrence of cortical breach [15, 66, 67]. To prevent this, Scolaro and colleagues introduced a novel technique using multiple percutaneously placed Poller-type Steinmann pins at the potential breaching site [66]. This strategy ensures safe passage of medullary reamers and femoral nails without causing a breach on the femoral cortex. Changing the nail entry from piriformis fossa laterally to the tip of greater trochanter will allow the nail to be fit in the bowed femurs, while also decreasing the danger of deformity and speeding up healing time. In the severely varus femur, using a the lateral entry for the straight nail may be a useful method [68].

There are several factors that cause iatrogenic fracture of the neck of the femur during antegrade intramedullary nailing. Impaction of the prominent edge of the nail to a valgus neck (cervicotrochanteric angle >135°), forced use of the bone awl instrument in the wrong direction, and multiple attempts to place the proximal locking screw accurately can all lead to fracture [12]. Patients on bisphosphonate therapy are at increased risk of iatrogenic fractures in other regions [69].

Subtrochanteric fractures are highly unstable fractures, often highly comminuted, make treatment difficult. When they are fixed with a proximal femoral nail, exact technical performance of implantation is the fundamental surgical prerequisite. The proximal constituent of the proximal femoral nail construct has two screws—a larger lag screw for load bearing, and a smaller hip screw for rotational stability. The lag screw has to be longer, preferably 10 mm longer than the hip screw, to avoid vertical forces and to prevent a knife effect or Z effect, thereby inducing the cut-out. This may force the hip screw to migrate into the joint and the lag screw to slide laterally [16, 51]. Although the Asian version of the proximal femoral nail is designed with a smaller diameter and other changes, it still creates inconvenience in fixation [51]. Hence, the surgeon needs to maintain accurate, painstaking, specialized surgical methodology.

The open interlocking nailing methodology had been studied in an Indian teaching institute, where it was concluded that it is a safe procedure for femoral shaft fractures [70]. It can be performed in the developing world with good functional and clinical results. It is advised in rural hospitals with no fracture table and image intensifier, in irreducible fractures, and in pregnant women [70]. A recent study compared open reduction with closed reduction in intramedullary femur fixation and showed similar results in rates of union, time of union, and complications for both methods [12].

When placing locking bolts, it is important to take good anteroposterior and lateral radiographs to ensure proper placement [71]. It has been reported that an antegrade titanium nail survives more than a million compression/bending cycles when the distal femur fracture is more than 3 cm from the more proximal of the two distal locking screws [62].

In the case of successive distal and periprosthetic proximal femoral fracture with compromised soft tissue, a novel "kissing nail technique" has been introduced for the exchange of intramedullary implants in adjacent peri-implant fractures. For the new proximal femur fracture, the tip of a distal femoral nail is advanced just until it passes the proximal fracture, thereby reducing both fractures, while an extra-long femoral nail 3 mm thicker than the existing distal femoral nail is passed and advanced distally. The long femoral nail is implanted in a "kissing nail" position, such that the tips of the two nails are touching each other and holding all fracture fragments in functional reduction. The distal femoral nail is then gradually pulled backward and fragment stability is maintained while both nails are past the distal fracture nonunion [72].

There is a noteworthy relation between pudendal nerve paralysis and comminuted femoral fractures [28]. Too much traction on the fracture table is considered to be a factor in producing pudendal nerve palsy during intramedullary nailing of the femur. Too much adduction of the hip or vigorous manipulation for reductions of the fracture will significantly increase the traction forces and should be avoided [73].

Intramedullary femoral devices should be avoided if the quantity or quality of bone is inadequate or the medullary canal is obliterated, or when faced a condition that may retard healing, blood supply limitations, active and previous infections, congenital or acquired bony deformity, hypovolemia, hypothermia, or coagulopathy. They must also be used cautiously in mentally challenged individuals who may not cooperate during rehabilitation [58].

Intramedullary nails used for fixation of femoral fractures can require removal for a variety of reasons. Nonmedically indicated implant removal must be avoided due to its high complication rate of 28%. Also, secondary fractures occur after implant removal in 27–44% of proximal fractures. Surgeons and patients must be aware of these imminent challenges and remove implants only for good medical reasons [74]. Even with a good medical reason, removal of an intact titanium femoral nail can be difficult and time-consuming. A third-generation conical, threaded extraction tool that was introduced in 2006 can make nail removal easier, faster, and safer, however [75].

McDonald and coworkers stressed the need of increased awareness with a high level of suspicion for the associated femoral shaft and neck fractures in any patient undergoing antegrade femoral nailing [62]. Preoperative radiography and CT scanning of the femoral neck and on-table plain radiographs should be performed as a routine practice, prior to the patient's recovering from anaesthesia and extubation [63].

Damage to the femoral vessels is a noted iatrogenic obstacle during surgery for intertrochanteric femur fractures. Such injuries commonly occur during procedures using short proximal femoral nails and dynamic hip screw. Procedures using long nails and their locking screws have fewer incidences of vascular injuries because of their distal relationship to the femoral vessels. The proximal femoral artery is much closer to the distal locking screw of the short nails [10].

Vascular injuries following hip fracture surgery can lead to limb dysfunction or even be life-threatening. Most vascular injuries (91.2%) are extrapelvic; intrapelvic injuries are less common (8.2%). The deep femoral artery is the most frequently injured vessel (78.3%), followed by the superficial femoral artery (10.8%). While drilling in the anterosuperior quadrant of the acetabulum for uncemented total hip replacement, one must take great care to prevent injury to the external iliac vein [27].

A complete vascular study both preoperatively and before the patient leaves the operating room is necessary to evaluate and diagnose any abnormalities in a controlled environment. When an unrecognized iatrogenic injury happens, several postoperative neurovascular investigations can help early recognition and corrective actions [76]. All through the treatment of femoral fractures, it is vital to be vigil and observe the signs of possible blood vessel damage. When a patient has acute pain and swelling in the middle thigh or inexplicable anemia in the postoperative period, the possibility that these symptoms may be due to an injury to the femoral vessels must be foremost in consideration [24].

To prevent vascular injuries and formation of pseudoaneurysm in femur surgery, it is recommended to release the traction and to position the patient in neutral position when inserting the distal screws for proximal femoral nailing. Further, cautious usage of the bone drill bit is advised. Excessive force should not be used when drilling to penetrate the medial cortex. Suitable drill guides should to be used to avoid overpenetration of the femur. Also, the screws should be precisely sized to penetrate the far cortex but no longer [10, 24].

Although elastic stable intramedullary nailing is the standard management of pediatric long bone fractures, there is reported 34–60% rate of complications after this procedure. Understanding the principles of this special surgery is vital in getting good results [45, 77, 78]. Vigilant preoperative planning to choose the appropriate-sized elastic nails and intraoperative studying of fracture stability under constant imaging after the operation are advised. It is recommended to palpate the nail end to avoid the nail being proud and also to confirm free motion of the knee joint following nail cutting and bending.

A 2017 study demonstrated that intravenous drug abuse, open fracture, and fracture comminution are independent predictors of nonunion and venous thromboembolism after intramedullary nailing of femoral diaphyseal fractures [79].

Some surgeons have reported high complication rates after LISS plating during the management of complex osteoporotic distal femur fractures. Use of intramedullary bone grafting (augmented LISS) resulted in significant increase of fracture stability under axial loading in comparison with conventional LISS plating [80].

Fractures of the femur after a knee or hip arthroplasty have been noted with high complication rates. The LISS system is an appropriate treatment option for such fractures associated with a stable hip or knee prosthesis [81].

LISS plating gives acceptable results in periprosthetic fractures after total knee replacement, but unsuccessful cases are on the rise. A recent study has indicated that reasons for failure include early weight bearing, obesity, osteoporosis, and lateral collateral ligament injury due to wrong plate placement [82]. These complications can be avoided by longer waiting period for weight bearing, active osteoporosis therapy, and intraoperative imaging to ensure the plate is positioned optimally [82].

Cerclage wire is another useful fracture fixation method. Its efficacy for treating femoral periprosthetic fractures, especially in the subtrochanteric region, has been demonstrated, because it allows femoral fixation even if there is a stem in the diaphysis. It securely holds the proximal femur with a supplementary plate. Recent advances in minimally invasive surgery with plate fixation have made it so the cerclage wire can be inserted percutaneously. However, its mechanical benefits can be compromised by local ischemia. There is a reported case of vascular complication after this percutaneous wiring procedure caused entire lower limb ischemia and eventually the death of the patient [83]. The presence of severe atherosclerosis is a sign of challenged tissue elasticity. This obstacle can be avoided by preparing the bone surfaces well and cautiously placing the patient on the fracture table to avoid forced adduction [2].

Damage control orthopaedics surgery with external fixation is safer as an initial approach for femoral shaft fracture in the multiply injured patient over early total care with intramedullary nailing. This approach considerably decreases the emergency operative time and blood loss [81]. Placement of external fixation pins and frames is an excellent minimally invasive method of establishing the stability of the bone and joints in the emergency setting of multiply severely injured patient. However, dangerous vascular complications can occur after femur shaft external fixation surgery [76]. While the surgeon must consider the safe zones for external fixator pins in the femur [66], the neurovascular structures will still be at risk because the normal regional anatomy is much altered in severe trauma. A vigilant examination of external fixator pin fixation is essential to avoid iatrogenic injury during damage control orthopaedic surgery [76].

Femoral shaft fractures in children are among the most common fractures that require hospitalization. The key deciding factor in treatment choice is the age of the child [84]. Fractures in children below 6 years of age can be managed nonoperatively with admirable outcomes. Elastic stable intramedullary nails are advised for children less than 11 years of age or those with body weight below 50 kg with a length stable transverse or short oblique fracture. Lengthy unstable fractures and fractures at the proximal ends of femur are to be treated by LISS plating or external fixation. For the children older than 11 with body weight above 50 kg, rigid intramedullary nailing or LISS plating is advised. As mentioned above, avoid having nail enter the piriformis fossa to prevent the risk of avascular necrosis of the femoral head [49].

Patients with hip and femur fractures may have comorbid factors that place them at high risk of complications and even death. Hence, surgeons should carefully assess the patients' preoperative status while counseling them on the risks of surgery [25, 85].

Excessive dissection and muscle stripping to place multiple fixation tools are to be avoided since they can produce delayed union or nonunion of fractures as a result of osseous devascularization. A recent meta-analysis advised that percutaneous reduction using special tools is a better choice than other reduction surgeries for management of femoral fractures [86].

Nonunion is a common challenge (23%) following intramedullary nailing of subtrochanteric fractures of the femur [2]. The intraoperative rectification of varus malalignment and re-establishment of the medial cortical support are the most significant risk factors for nonunion after such surgery. The surgeon must watch for autodynamization (early breakage or loosening of distal locking screws) of the nail within the initial 3 months of surgery, which is a good predictor of malfunction and which may lead to revision surgery [2].

Some surgeons still use the Küntscher nail (K-nail) for selective cases of simple transverse, short oblique midshaft diaphyseal femur fractures. There is a recent report on spontaneous distal migration and protrusion of a K-nail with infective complication in India [87]. It is highly advised that these nails be removed as soon as radiologic union and consolidation of the fracture is established to avoid the distal migration of the nail.

There is a 6% incidence of infection in femur fracture surgery [88]. It is highly recommended that all health establishments implement an antibiotic stewardship program and safety protocols to prevent and manage surgical site infections [13, 55, 89–93] (see also Chap. 1).

The orthopaedic surgeon must recognize that fractures change anatomic landmarks. The safe zones may disappear because of fracture fragment movement. Awareness of all the technical alternatives to fracture fixation is important [83]. The surgeon must also keep in mind that various iatrogenic complications can occur at all stages of instrumentation and must therefore be vigilant and respect all steps of the procedure, with gentle handling techniques. Complications can be well prevented and efficiently treated by thorough preoperative evaluation and cautious examination [14, 94].

References

1. Wang A, Zong S, Su L et al (2016) Meta-analysis of postoperative complications in distal femoral fractures: retrograde intramedullary nailing versus plating. *Int J Clin Exp Med* 9(10):18900–18911
2. Krappinger D, Wolf B, Dammerer D et al (2019) Risk factors for nonunion after intramedullary nailing of subtrochanteric femoral fractures. *Arch Orthop Trauma Surg* 139(6):769–777
3. Jose AK, Kumar S (2015) Titanium proximal femoral nailing for inter-trochanteric fractures of femur. *Int J Med Res* 3(9):990–995
4. Alobaidi AS, Al-Hassani A, El-Menyar A et al (2016) Early and late intramedullary nailing of femur fracture: a single center experience. *Int J Crit Illn Inj Sci* 6(3):143–147
5. Abraham VT, Chandrasekaran M, Mahapatra S (2016) Outcome of subtrochanteric fracture of the femur managed with proximal femoral nail. *Int Surg J* 3(3):1296–1300
6. Arora S, Mittal S, Aggarwal V et al (2013) Femoral artery thrombosis after closed femoral nailing: an unusual complication. *Orthop Surg* 5(1):68–71
7. Georgiannos D, Lampridis V, Bisbinas I (2014) Complications following treatment of trochanteric fractures with the Gamma3 Nail: is the latest version of Gamma Nail superior to its predecessor? *Surg Res Pract* 2014:143598
8. Neubauer T, Grechenig S, Leitner L et al (2016) Vascular complications in plating of the proximal femur: review. *Arch Orthop Trauma Surg* 136(4):539–551
9. Segal D, Yaacobi E, Marom N et al (2017) The incidence of life-threatening iatrogenic vessel injury following closed or open reduction and internal fixation of intertrochanteric femoral fractures. *Int Orthop* 41(9):1845–1850
10. Voorde KV, Dauwe J, Van Oost J (2018) Late presentation of an iatrogenic pseudoaneurysm of the profunda femoris artery following intramedullary nailing. *Case Rep Orthop* 2018:8270256
11. Labronici PJ, Dos Santos Filho FC, Diamantino YLO et al (2019) Proximal femur fracture and vascular injury in adults: case report. *Rev Bras Ortop (Sao Paulo)* 54(3):343–346
12. Telgheder ZL, Albanese MA, Bloom DS et al (2020) A comparison of complications and union rates in intramedullary nailing of femoral shaft fractures treated with open versus closed reduction. *Orthopedics* 43(2):103–107

13. World Health Organization. Antimicrobial stewardship programmes in health-care facilities in low- and middle-income countries: a WHO practical toolkit. Published 2019. https://apps.who.int/iris/handle/10665/329404
14. Deshpande M, Shanmugam K, Fadte K (2019) Proximal femoral nailing—intra operative complications: a retrospective analysis of 200 cases of proximal femoral fractures. *Int J Orthop Sci* 5(2):985–990
15. Chopra BL, Kumar K, Khajotia BL et al (2017) Proximal femoral nail outcome and complications: a prospective study of 125 cases of proximal femoral fractures. *Int J Res Orthop* 3(5):973–978
16. Mavrogenis AF, Panagopoulos GN, Megaloikonomos PD et al (2016) Complications after hip nailing for fractures. *Orthopedics* 39(1):e108–e116
17. Chen H-W, Pan J (2017) Reverse LISS plate in treating femoral intertrochanteric fractures: a review of 22 cases. *Biomed Res* 28(7)
18. Zelle BA, Webb AJ, Matson C et al (2018) Safety and efficacy of a two-screw cephalomedullary nail for intertrochanteric femur fracture fixation: a retrospective case series in 264 patients. *Patient Saf Surg* 12:31
19. Akshay TM, Naganagoudar IH (2015) A clinical study on intra-operative and delayed complication in surgical management following peri-trochanteric fracture using proximal femoral nail. *Med Innov (Online)* 4(2):29–34
20. Karanikas I, Lazarides M, Arvanitis D et al (1993) Iatrogenic arterial trauma associated with hip fracture surgery. *Acta Chir Belg* 93(6):284–286
21. Mehta V, Finn HA (2005) Femoral artery and vein injury after cerclage wiring of the femur: a case report. *J Arthroplasty* 20(6):811–814
22. Bansal R, Laing PW (2006) Iatrogenic blunt arterial injury during a hip fracture surgery. *Acta Orthop Belg* 72(1):96–99
23. Kadzielski J, Vrahas M (2010) A vascular complication of trochanteric–entry femoral nailing on a fracture table. *Am J Orthop (Nelle Mead NJ)* 39(7):E64–E66
24. Yoon HK, Oh HC, Park J et al (2016) Rupture of the deep femoral artery during proximal femoral nailing following an intertrochanteric fracture: a case report. *Hip Pelvis* 28(1):54–59
25. Siddiqui YS, Naqvi SEH, Sherwani MKA, Ahmad A (2019) Vascular complication following total hip replacement: a nightmare for arthroplasty surgeon. *MOJ Orthop Rheumatol* 11(5):183–186
26. Bråten M, Helland P, Myhre HO et al (1996) 11 femoral fractures with vascular injury: good outcome with early vascular repair and internal fixation. *Acta Orthop Scand* 67(2):161–164
27. Müdüroglu A, Kayhan TO, Yüksel A (2017) Iliac vein injury during total hip replacement: a rare iatrogenic complication and its successful surgical treatment. *Int J Vasc Surg Med* 3(2):033–035
28. Rose R, Chang S, Felix R et al (2007) Pudendal nerve palsy following static intramedullary nailing of the femur. Internet J Orthop Surg 10(1) spub.com/IJOS/10/1/11059
29. Siddiqui YS, Khan AQ, Asif N et al (2019) Modes of failure of proximal femoral nail (PFN) in unstable trochanteric fractures. *MOJ Orthop Rheumatol* 11(1):7–16
30. Bråten M, Terjesen T, Rossvoll I (1995) Femoral shaft fractures treated by intramedullary nailing: a follow-up study focusing on problems related to the method. *Injury* 26(6):379–383
31. Raasck K, Al FH (2018) The effects of simultaneous versus staged bilateral femoral intramedullary nailing for metastatic disease on survival time and perioperative complications: a systematic review. *J Orthop Oncol* 4(2):125
32. Khan FA, Ikram MA, Badr AA, al-Khawashki H (1995) Femoral neck fracture: a complication of femoral nailing. *Injury* 26(5):319–321
33. Moghtadaei M, Otoukesh B, Kaghazian P et al (2016) Risk of superior gluteal nerve injury after using ante-grade femoral nailing. *Biomed Pharmacol J* 9(1):419–424
34. Saikia KC, Bhuyan SK, Bhattacharya TD, Saikia SP (2007) Titanium elastic nailing in femoral diaphyseal fractures of children in 6-16 years of age. *Indian J Orthop* 41(4):381–385

35. Singh P, Kumar R (2012) Pediatric femoral shaft fracture management by titanium elastic nailing; a prospective study of 112 patients. Internet J Orthop Surg 19(3) http://ispub.com/IJOS/19/3/14336
36. Lascombes P, Nespola A, Poircuitte J-M et al (2012) Early complications with flexible intramedullary nailing in childhood fracture: 100 cases managed with precurved tip and shaft nails. *Orthop Traumatol Surg Res* 98(4):369–375
37. Chincholi S (2016) Management of paediatric femoral shaft fractures with titanium elastic nails. *Int J Orthop Sci* 2(4):106–108
38. Govindasamy R, Gnanasundaram R, Kasirajan S et al (2018) Elastic stable intramedullary nailing of femoral shaft fracture: experience in 48 children. *Arch Bone Jt Surg* 6(1):39–46
39. Kawalkar A, Badole CM (2018) Percutaneous titanium elastic nail for femoral shaft fracture in patient between 5 and 15 years. *J Orthop* 15(2):695–700
40. Hwaizi LJ, Saeed AMS, Mahmood MN (2018) Diaphyseal femoral fractures in children: comparison between elastic stable intramedullary nailing and conservative management. *Open Orthop J* 12:435–444
41. May C, Yen Y-M, Nasreddine AY et al (2013) Complications of plate fixation of femoral shaft fractures in children and adolescents. *J Child Orthop* 7(3):235–243
42. Canavese F, Marengo L, Andreacchio A et al (2016) Complications of elastic stable intramedullary nailing of femoral shaft fractures in children weighing fifty kilograms (one hundred and ten pounds) and more. *Int Orthop* 40(12):2627–2634
43. Piétu G, Ehlinger M (2017) Minimally invasive internal fixation of distal femur fractures. *Orthop Traumatol Surg Res* 103(1S):S161–S169
44. Schandelmaier P, Krettek C, Miclau T et al (1999) Stabilization of distal femoral fractures using the LISS. *Tech Orthop*:230–246
45. Kanabar P, Kumar V, Owen PJ, Rushton N (2007) Less invasive stabilisation system plating for distal femoral fractures. *J Orthop Surg (Hong Kong)* 15(3):299–302
46. Kow RY, Low CL, Jaya Raj J et al (2019) Heterotopic ossification of the hip post reamed intramedullary femoral nail: a case report. *Orthop Res Online J* 5(4):OPROJ.000619.2019
47. Tuttle MS, Smith WR, Williams AE et al (2009) Safety and efficacy of damage control external fixation versus early definitive stabilization for femoral shaft fractures in the multiple-injured patient. *J Trauma* 67(3):602–605
48. Dissaneewate P, Apivatthakakul T (2019) Safe zone for placement of anterior distal femoral half pins. J Med Assoc Thai 102(3):343–346
49. John R, Sharma S, Raj GN et al (2017) Current concepts in paediatric femoral shaft fractures. *Open Orthop J* 11:353–368
50. Hoppenfeld S, de Boer P, Buckley R (2022) *Surgical exposures in orthopaedics: the anatomic approach*, 6th edn. Wolters Kluwer, Philadelphia
51. Kanthimathi B, Narayanan VI (2012) Early complications in proximal femoral nailing done for treatment of subtrochanteric fractures. *Malays Orthop J* 6(1):25–29
52. Beltran MJ, Collinge CA, Patzkowski JC et al (2012) The safe zone for external fixator pins in the femur. *J Orthop Trauma* 26(11):643–647
53. Hossain MM, Alam QS, Haque E, Rahman MS (2014) Management of fracture shaft of femur in children with titanium elastic nailing (TEN) at Dhaka Medical College Hospital, Bangladesh. *J Dhaka Med Coll* 23(1):24–30
54. Khalifa AA, Ahmed AM, Khaled M, Said EA (2019) Factors contributing to superior gluteal nerve injury during cephalomedullary nailing of femoral fractures. *J Orthop Allied Sci* 7(1):4–7
55. National Institute for Health and Care Excellence. Open fractures in hospital. NICE Pathways. Published 2021. https://pathways.nice.org.uk/pathways/trauma/open-fractures-in-hospital
56. Asadollahi S, Holcdorf D, Stella DL, Bucknill A (2020) Identification of the lateral femoral safe zone for drilling during LISS plate fixation of distal femur fractures. *Injury* 51(2):452–456
57. Piponov H, Osmani FA, Parekh A et al (2021) A novel method for predicting superior gluteal nerve safe zones in the lateral approach to the hip. *Clin Anat* 34(4):522–526

58. Smith & Nephew. Intramedullary nail system: important medical information. Issued 2010. https://www.smith-nephew.com/global/assets/pdf/products/surgical/im%20nails%20(english)%2081068703%20b%202010-02.pdf
59. Papachristos IV (2019) Complications of femoral intramedullary nailing: what should the surgeon remember? *EC Orthopaedics* 10(6):477–482
60. Hwang SK, Yoon JS (1990) Pitfalls and complications in the use of interlocking intramedullary nailing for the femoral fractures. *J Korean Soc Fract* 3(1):71–78
61. Castellanos J, Garcia-Nuño L, Cavanilles-Walker JM, Roca J (2009) Iatrogenic femoral neck fracture during closed nailing of the femoral shaft fracture. *Eur J Trauma Emerg Surg* 35(5):479–481
62. Karadimas EJ, Papadimitriou G, Theodoratos G et al (2009) The effectiveness of the antegrade reamed technique: the experience and complications from 415 traumatic femoral shaft fractures. *Strategies Trauma Limb Reconstr* 4(3):113–121
63. McDonald LS, Tepolt F, Leonardelli D et al (2013) A cascade of preventable complications following a missed femoral neck fracture after antegrade femoral nailing. *Patient Saf Surg* 7:16
64. Antekeier SB, Burden RL Jr, Voor MJ, Roberts CS (2005) Mechanical study of the safe distance between distal femoral fracture site and distal locking screws in antegrade intramedullary nailing. *J Orthop Trauma* 19(10):693–697
65. Lakhwani OP (2012) Correlation of trochanter–shaft angle in selection of entry site in antegrade intramedullary femoral nail. *ISRN Orthop* 2012:431374
66. Scolaro JA, Endress C, Mehta S (2013) Prevention of cortical breach during placement of an antegrade intramedullary femoral nail. *Orthopedics* 36(9):688–692
67. Fantry AJ, Elia G, Vopat BG, Daniels AH (2015) Distal femoral complications following antegrade intramedullary nail placement. *Orthop Rev (Pavia)* 7(1):5820
68. Kim JW, Kim H, Oh C-W et al (2017) Surgical outcomes of intramedullary nailing for diaphyseal atypical femur fractures: is it safe to modify a nail entry in bowed femur? *Arch Orthop Trauma Surg* 137(11):1515–1522
69. Barimani B, Khan K, Abduljabbar F et al (2020) Unexpected iatrogenic fracture of the femoral neck during subtrochanteric fracture fixation in a patient on bisphosphonate treatment for osteoporosis: case report. *Trauma Case Rep* 26:100290
70. Manjhi LB, Suman SK, Kumar R, Singh SKK (2017) Open interlocking nailing of the fracture of the shaft of femur. *Int J Orthop Sci* 3(2):611–613
71. Kyle RF. Treating femoral fractures with intramedullary rods is safe but tricky. *Healio Orthopedics Today*. April 1, 2010. https://www.healio.com/news/orthopedics/20120325/treating-femoral-fractures-with-intramedullary-rods-is-safe-but-tricky
72. Melcher C, Delhey PR, Birkenmaier C, Thaller PH (2017) "Kissing nail technique" for the exchange of intramedullary implants in adjacent peri-implant fractures. *Acta Orthop Traumatol Turc* 51(6):488–491
73. Brumback RJ, Ellison TS, Molligan H et al (1992) Pudendal nerve palsy complicating intramedullary nailing of the femur. *J Bone Joint Surg Am* 74(10):1450–1455
74. Kovar FM, Strasser E, Jaindl M et al (2015) Complications following implant removal in patients with proximal femur fractures: an observational study over 16 years. *Orthop Traumatol Surg Res* 101(7):785–789
75. Wood GW II (2006) Safe, rapid, and effortless femoral nail removal using a new third-generation universal femoral nail extraction tool. *J Orthop Sci* 11(6):626–627
76. Staeheli GR, Fraser MR, Morgan SJ (2012) The dangers of damage control orthopedics: a case report of vascular injury after femoral fracture external fixation. *Patient Saf Surg* 6:7
77. Nisar A, Bhosale A, Madan SS et al (2013) Complications of elastic stable intramedullary nailing for treating paediatric long bone fractures. *J Orthop* 10(1):17–24
78. Salonen A, Lahdes-Vasama T, Mattila VM et al (2015) Pitfalls of femoral titanium elastic nailing. *Scand J Surg* 104(2):121–126
79. Clement ND, Beresford-Cleary NJA, Simpson AHRW (2017) Femoral diaphyseal fractures in young adults: predictors of complications. *Arch Trauma Res* 6(3):20–24

80. Todorov D, Zderic I, Richards RG et al (2018) Is augmented LISS plating biomechanically advantageous over conventional LISS plating in unstable osteoporotic distal femoral fractures? *J Orthop Res* 36(10):2604–2611
81. O'Toole RV, Gobezie R, Hwang R et al (2006) Low complication rate of LISS for femur fractures adjacent to stable hip or knee arthroplasty. *Clin Orthop Relat Res* 450:203–210
82. Tian Z-J, Liu Y-J, Chen B-J et al (2020) Failure of less-invasive stabilization system (LISS) plating for periprosthetic distal femur fractures: three case reports. *Medicine (Baltimore)* 99(8):e19195
83. Ehlinger M, Niglis L, Favreau H et al (2018) Vascular complication after percutaneous femoral cerclage wire. *Orthop Traumatol Surg Res* 104(3):377–381
84. Montreal Children's Hospital. Intramedullary nailing for femur fracture management: a guide for parents. McGill University Health Center. Published 2016. https://www.thechildren.com/sites/default/files/PDFs/Trauma/LatestUpdates/intramedullary_nailing_for_femur_fracture_web_version_english.pdf
85. Horner NS, Samuelsson K, Solyom J et al (2017) Implant-related complications and mortality after use of short and long gamma nail for intertrochanteric and subtrochanteric fractures: a prospective study with minimum 13-year follow-up. *JB JS Open Access* 2(3):e0026
86. Zhu T, Qiu S, Li N et al (2018) The effect of percutaneous reduction during intramedullary nailing for femoral and tibial fractures: a meta-analysis. *Int J Clin Exp Med* 11(5):5367–5374
87. Jain S, Nag HL, Kantiwal P, Hulmani D (2020) Spontaneous distal migration and protrusion of a Küntscher intramedullary nail from the left femur: a rare complication. *Cureus* 12(1):e6576
88. Young S, Banza LN, Hallan G et al (2013) Complications after intramedullary nailing of femoral fractures in a low-income country. *Acta Orthop* 84(5):460–467
89. National Institute for Health and Care Excellence. Antimicrobial stewardship: systems and processes for effective antimicrobial medicine use. NICE guideline 15. Published August 18, 2015. https://www.nice.org.uk/guidance/ng15
90. World Alliance for Patient Safety. Safe surgery saves lives: the second global safety challenge. World Health Organization website. Published 2009. https://www.who.int/patientsafety/safesurgery/knowledge_base/SSSL_Brochure_finalJun08.pdf
91. Seligman KM, Katz D, Farber MK (2018) Preventing surgical site infection after cesarean delivery: the anesthesia professional's role. *APSF Newsletter* 33(1):25–27
92. National Institute for Health and Care Excellence. Surgical site infections: prevention and treatment. NICE guideline 125. Published 2020. https://www.nice.org.uk/guidance/ng125
93. Farooqui HH, Mehta A, Selvaraj S (2019) Outpatient antibiotic prescription rate and pattern in the private sector in India: evidence from medical audit data. *PLoS One* 14(11):e0224848
94. Bouya A, Elghoul N, Zaddoug O et al (2019) Iatrogenic femoral neck fracture: an unusual cause. *Int J Res Orthop* 5(5):961–964

Safe Knee Surgery 11

11.1 Introduction

Most diseases and fractures of the knee are amenable to surgical treatment. Despite the progress that has been made in implants and techniques of knee surgery, considerable complications still occur [1], many of which are preventable [2].

Total knee replacement is a safe, cost-effective treatment for lessening pain and restoring function in patients with knee degeneration who are not responding to conservative mode of therapy. It is a widely performed procedure all over the world with a high rate of patient satisfaction. Despite this, complications do occur and can cause major morbidity. Although neurovascular complications are infrequent in knee surgery, their occurrence can be potentially disastrous for the affected lower limb [3, 4]. It is the responsibility of the surgeon to be aware of such risks in order to inform the patient preoperatively and to promptly respond to complications during surgery and in the postoperative period [1].

Distal femoral fractures are managed with the less-invasive stabilization system (LISS) or distal femoral nailing. With appropriate application, distal femoral nailing is acceptable for all fractures of the distal third of the femoral shaft, including highly unstable bicondylar fractures, and does not cause damage to the soft tissues the knee joint [5]. There are no differences in outcome and complications with LISS and distal femoral nailing in treating distal femoral fractures [6].

The treatment of selected osteoporotic complex intra-articular fractures of the proximal tibia with compression bolts and intramedullary nailing offers particular advantages. In these types of fractures of the proximal tibia, treatment results based on the type of fracture as well as good treatment. When accurate alignment, joint stability, and perfect articular surfaces are achieved, the outcomes are very good [7, 8].

S. V. Babu, *Safe Orthopaedic Surgery*,
https://doi.org/10.1007/978-981-16-2846-7_11

11.2 Principles of Safe Knee Surgery [1, 9–16]

11.2.1 Safety Principles for Arthroscopic Surgery of the Knee

- The articular cartilage in the knee joint can be injured at two phases during arthroscopy—while incising or by forceful placement of the arthroscope. If the incision is made cautiously, this problem will not occur. If resistance is met when manipulating the scope within the knee, it is a sign that the articular cartilage is being encountered.
- More posteriorly placed incisions on the medial side can damage the articular surface of the medial femoral condyle. Therefore, it is recommended that more posteromedial or posterolateral incisions be made under direct arthroscopic control.
- The meniscus can be damaged by the surgical knife or by the scope if the incisions are made very close to the line of knee joint.
- Flexion of the knee to 90° (the "figure of four" position) must be used as the arthroscopic instruments are approaching the posterolateral corner of the knee to decrease the risk of nerve injury in cases of capsular infiltration, since the neurovascular structures are farther from the knee capsule in this position (Fig. 11.1).

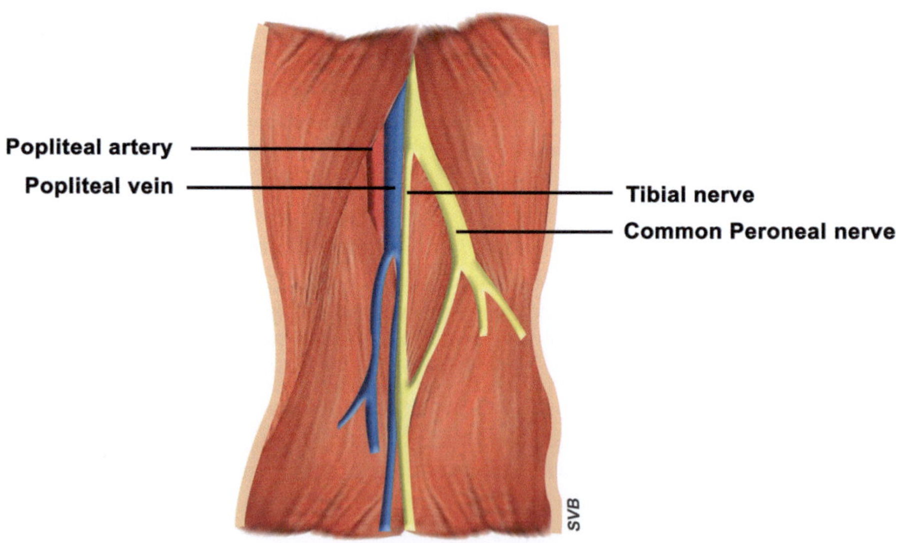

Fig. 11.1 The knee and its neurovascular relations (posterior aspect)

11.2.2 Safety Principles for the Medial Parapatellar Approach to the Knee

- The infrapatellar branch of the saphenous nerve is commonly injured during this approach.
- The patellar ligament has to be handled very gently, since the ligament is difficult to reattach if it becomes avulsed from its insertion on the tibia.

11.2.3 Safety Principles for Medial Meniscectomy of the Knee

- The infrapatellar branch of the saphenous nerve may be injured if the incision is placed more than 1 cm below the joint line.
- The popliteal artery is just behind the posterior joint capsule. Any injury here will damage the artery. If the knee is flexed, this portion of the joint capsule detaches from the tibia and femur, taking the artery along with it.
- The coronary ligament (the meniscotibial element of the deep medial ligament) attaches the periphery of the meniscus to the joint capsule and tibia, and may get damaged if the incision through the synovium is made along the joint line.
- Incisions done more posteriorly may injure the superficial medial ligament (the tibial collateral ligament) as it goes from the medial epicondyle of the femur to its insertion on the tibia just below the pes anserinus.
- The fat pad occupies significant amounts of the anterior portion of the knee joint and must not be damaged. Injury will produce adhesions within the joint and may compromise the blood supply of the patella.
- The medial meniscus may be incised by accident during the opening of the synovium. This can be prevented by entering the knee joint well above the joint line.

11.2.4 Safety Principles for the Medial Approach to the Knee and Its Supporting Structures

- The saphenous nerve arises between the gracilis and sartorius muscles and runs with the long saphenous vein. It supplies some of the non-weight-bearing portions of the foot and should be safeguarded.
- The saphenous vein is seen in the posterior corner of the knee during superficial dissection.
- The medial inferior genicular artery curves around the superior portion of the tibia. It may be injured when the medial head of gastrocnemius muscle is lifted off the posterior capsule.

- The popliteal artery is present on the posterior joint capsule in the midline and is near to the medial head of the gastrocnemius muscle. Utmost care must be taken to prevent injuring the vessel during dissection of the gastrocnemius from the joint capsule.

11.2.5 Safety Principles for Lateral Meniscectomy of the Knee

- The lateral meniscus will be damaged if the synovium is incised too close to the joint line.
- The lateral inferior genicular artery goes around the upper part of the tibia. The artery is present near to the peripheral attachment of the lateral meniscus; it may be injured if the meniscus is removed along with a portion of the capsule during meniscectomy, leading to massive hemarthrosis.
- If the superficial lateral ligament (fibular collateral ligament) is injured and not reconstructed, it may lead to lateral instability.

11.2.6 Safety Principles for the Lateral Approach to the Knee

- The common peroneal nerve is the highly potential structure to get injured during this approach. It present on the posterior border of the biceps tendon and should be found early in this procedure, as the supporting structures of the lateral side of the knee getting dissected, the nerve has to be seen and protected well.
- The lateral superior genicular artery goes in between the lateral head of the gastrocnemius muscle and the posterolateral capsule. It requires ligation for full exposure of the posterolateral corner.
- The popliteus tendon is in danger as it travels within the joint before it reaches to the posterior aspect of the meniscus and the femur. While opening the posterior half of the knee joint capsule, we need to take care to prevent cutting the tendon.
- The lateral meniscus or its coronary ligament may be incised by chance, if arthrotomy is done very close to the joint line.

11.2.7 Safety Principles for the Posterior Approach to the Knee

- The medial sural cutaneous nerve, which is present lateral to the small saphenous vein, may be injured as it travels below the deep fascia of the calf. Incising the deep fascia of the calf muscle just medial to the vein will safeguard the nerve.
- The tibial nerve may be damaged in the popliteal fossa, and the common peroneal nerve also is vulnerable to damage in the popliteal fossa, so much care has to be given when dissecting.
- The small saphenous vein and popliteal vessels may get injured during the deeper surgery.

11.2.8 Safety Principles for the Lateral Approach to the Distal Femur for Anterior Cruciate Ligament Surgery

- The peroneal nerve may be damaged if the surgical plane is losing its way out of the posterior region of the biceps femoris muscle.
- The lateral superior genicular artery is to be safeguarded while incising.
- The popliteal artery will be damaged if the surgical dissection does not remain subperiosteal. When the intercondylar notch is felt, the knee has to be flexed to 90° to make the popliteal artery fall posteriorly within the joint capsule.

11.2.9 Safety Principles for Minimally Invasive Surgical Approaches of LISS, Nailing, and Knee Replacement Surgery

- The minimally invasive approaches for extra- and intra-articular distal femoral fractures are not the same.
  - For extra-articular fractures, a skin incision is made from Gerdy's tubercle about 80 mm in proximal direction. Then, the iliotibial tract is directed in the direction of the fibers. The interval between the lateral vastus and the periosteum is opened. Distally, the lateral vastus muscle inserts mainly on the femoral ridge. There are no major muscle insertions on the lateral periosteum or bone. The internal fixator of the LISS can be inserted in the plane between the periosteum and the muscle.
  - For intra-articular fractures, an anterolateral arthrotomy giving good control of the reduction is advised. This arthrotomy also permits a subsequent introduction of the LISS fixator and allows the lag screws to be fixed from medially.

- The most common errors in LISS while treating distal femoral fractures are related to insufficient reduction of the fracture. Proper use of intraoperative imaging and correct application of the principles of LISS as advised by the manufacturer will yield excellent results.
- There are several minimally invasive surgical techniques for knee replacement surgery that will reduce quadriceps damage and also prevent patellar eversion.
  - The mini arthrotomy procedure uses a smaller sized arthrotomy than a traditional medial parapatellar arthrotomy.
  - The mini mid-vastus technique has an incision that extends 2 cm or more into the vastus medialis muscle.
  - The medial quad-sparing approach uses a more medially placed incision and avoids a quadriceps sparing arthrotomy.
  - The direct lateral approach uses an 8- to 10-cm incision from below Gerdy's tubercle to the lateral epicondyle lateral to the patella.

- The best entry point for retrograde femoral nailing is 1.2 cm anterior to the femoral origin of the posterior cruciate ligament. It is centered in the intercondylar sulcus to provides the most favorable balance of fracture reduction and knee joint sparing. It may be difficult to target this site with a percutaneous technique and will require direct visualization of the intercondylar sulcus for ideal nail placement.

11.3 Discussion

Since its inception, arthroscopy has been considered a standard and safe procedure in diagnosis and management of many conditions of knee, with fewer complications than open procedures and a low incidence of infection. However, the latest reports on knee arthroscopy show its overall complications are rising, with an incidence between 0.27% and 4.7% [3, 4, 17]. Major iatrogenic vascular trauma causing severe morbidity has been reported [4]. The meniscus is more susceptible to vascular injuries than other ligaments during arthroscopic surgery, and a high index of suspicion is warranted, with immediate treatment in these injuries [3, 4, 17].

The typical valgus and varus bending system of the knee in a lateral or medial plateau split fracture causes varying degrees of articular surface depression. This position leads to axis malalignment and pathologic load distribution, which ultimately cause poor functional outcome and posttraumatic osteoarthritis [18]. Associated ligament disruption or meniscus or cartilage damage can further worsen clinical results. Nonoperative treatment may be considered for nondisplaced intra-articular fractures of the lateral tibial condyle. Intra-articular joint displacement of more than 2 mm, metaphyseal-diaphyseal translation greater than 1 cm, lateral tilting of the plateau of more than 5°, condylar widening beyond 5 mm, angular deformity of more than 10° in either the coronal (varus–valgus) or the sagittal plane (tibial slope), associated compartment syndrome, associated ligamental injury requiring repair, associated fractures of the ipsilateral tibia or fibula, open fractures, and all fractures of the medial condyle should be reduced and fixed operatively [19]. In complex high-energy proximal tibial fractures involving the metadiaphyseal segment, restoration of the limb axis and length, accurate intra-articular reduction, and further avoidance of soft tissue injury are the most crucial elements. These fractures are associated with extensive soft tissue damage even in closed fractures. The management requires exemplary soft tissue handling and fine fracture reduction skills to prevent iatrogenic complications [13, 20].

Accurate anatomic reduction of the knee articular surface, re-establishment of functional anatomy, and stable fixation are compulsory for optimal knee function after distal femoral fractures. Failure to achieve these points because of the pattern of the fracture or inappropriate fixation will be followed by major functional discrepancy, slowing the patient's recovery [21].

The mortality rate of total knee replacement has been reported to be higher at low-volume institutions than at high-volume institutions (0.73% vs 0.43%) [1, 22]. Around 0.5–12% of patients who have knee replacement develop deep infection around the prosthesis [1, 22]. Periprosthetic infection can be life-changing for patients [22, 23], and there is a need for greater support throughout treatment and prolonged recovery. It is highly recommended that all health establishments implement an antibiotic stewardship program and safety protocols to prevent and manage surgical site infections [10, 11, 13–16, 22] (see also Chap. 1).

Cemented total knee replacement using a conventional medial parapatellar approach without computer navigation is the gold standard of knee replacement [1]. The advantages of minimally invasive surgery in total knee replacement are professed to be improved wound cosmesis, quicker recovery time, decreased length of hospital stay, and better function compared to the standard approach. A substantial learning curve accompanies minimally invasive techniques, however, which may be unacceptably long for surgeons performing low volumes of knee replacement surgery.

Although the incidence of nerve injuries following knee surgeries is low, they are more common in the diabetic population. The incidence of neurovascular injury after total knee replacement has been reported between 0.9% and 1.3% [1, 24, 25]. The common peroneal nerve injury is the most frequently injured nerve in knee arthroplasty and arthroscopy, and the saphenous nerve may be injured significantly during arthroscopy (0.3–10%) [1, 24, 25]. Possible mechanisms of iatrogenic nerve injury include nerve puncture, sutures tied over the nerve, capturing the nerve, and placing tension over the nerve, and nerve tethering. Orthopaedic surgeons should be aware that all kind of complications, including neurovascular and other vital structure injuries, could occur after knee surgery and should be able to recognize their clinical appearance immediately and begin prompt treatment. Medicolegally, the identified negligence is frequently the faulty treatment of the paralysis postoperatively, rather than the actual occurrence of the nerve injury [1, 24, 25].

References

1. Cheung A, Goh SK, Tang A, Keng TB (2008) Complications of total knee arthroplasty. *Curr Orthop* 22(4):274–283
2. Kim TK, Savino RM, McFarland EG, Cosgarea AJ (2002) Neurovascular complications of knee arthroscopy. *Am J Sports Med* 30(4):619–629
3. Neagoe RM, Bancu S, Muresan M, Sala D (2015) Major vascular injuries complicating knee arthroscopy. *Wideochir Inne Tech Maloinwazyjne* 10(2):266–274
4. Bernardi G, Tudisco C (2017) Transient common peroneal and tibial nerve palsy following knee arthroscopy for the treatment of discoid lateral meniscus. *Joints* 5(2):118–120
5. Grass R, Biewener A, Rammelt S, Zwipp H et al (2002) Retrograde locking nail osteosynthesis of distal femoral fractures with the distal femoral n ail (DFN) [article in German]. *Unfallchirurg* 105(4):298–314
6. Markmiller M, Konrad G, Südkamp N (2004) Femur-LISS and distal femoral nail for fixation of distal femoral fractures: are there differences in outcome and complications? *Clin Orthop Relat Res* 426:252–257
7. Pasa L, Kelbl M, Suchomel R et al (2007) Treatment of intra-articular proximal tibial evaluation of two- to seven-year follow-up [article in Czech]. *Acta Chir Orthop Traumatol Cech* 74(5):336–341

8. Garnavos C, Lasanianos NG (2011) The management of complex fractures of the proximal tibia with minimal intra-articular impaction in fragility patients using intramedullary nailing and compression bolts. *Injury* 42(10):1066–1072
9. Krupp RJ, Malkani AL, Goodin RA, Voor MJ (2003) Optimal entry point for retrograde femoral nailing. *J Orthop Trauma* 17(2):100–105
10. Hoppenfeld S, de Boer P, Buckley R (2022) *Surgical exposures in orthopaedics: the anatomic approach*, 6th edn. Wolters Kluwer, Philadelphia
11. World Alliance for Patient Safety. Safe surgery saves lives: the second global safety challenge. World Health Organization website. Published 2009. https://www.who.int/patientsafety/safesurgery/knowledge_base/SSSL_Brochure_finalJun08.pdf
12. National Institute for Health and Care Excellence. Antimicrobial stewardship: systems and processes for effective antimicrobial medicine use. NICE guideline 15. Published August 18, 2015. https://www.nice.org.uk/guidance/ng15
13. Wu D, Reng G, Shrivastava A et al (2015) A useful surgical strategy for proximal tibial fractures (AO/OTA type 41-C) with diaphyseal involvement. *Int J Clin Exp Med* 8(8):13455–13463
14. Seligman KM, Katz D, Farber MK (2018) Preventing surgical site infection after cesarean delivery: the anesthesia professional's role. *APSF Newsletter* 33(1):25–27
15. National Institute for Health and Care Excellence. Surgical site infections: prevention and treatment. NICE guideline 125. Published 2020. https://www.nice.org.uk/guidance/ng125
16. World Health Organization. Antimicrobial stewardship programmes in health-care facilities in low- and middle-income countries: a WHO practical toolkit. Published 2019. https://apps.who.int/iris/handle/10665/329404
17. Reigstad O, Grimsgaard C (2006) Complications in knee arthroscopy. *Knee Surg Sports Traumatol Arthrosc* 14(5):473–477
18. Aurich M, Koenig V, Hofmann G (2018) Communited intraarticular fractures of the tibial plateau lead to posttraumatic osteoarthritis of the knee: current treatment review. *Asian J Surg* 41(2):99–105
19. Raschke MJ, Kittl C, Domnick C (2017) Proximal tibia fractures. *EFORT Open Rev* 2(5):241–249
20. Khatri K, Sharma V, Goyal D, Farooque K (2016) Complications in the management of closed high-energy proximal tibial plateau fractures. *Chin J Traumatol* 19:342–347
21. Lupescu O, Nagea M, Patru C et al (2015) Treatment options for distal femoral fractures. *Maedica (Bucur)* 10(2):117–122
22. Mallon CM, Gooberman-Hill R, Moore AJ (2018) Infection after knee replacement: a qualitative study of impact of periprosthetic knee infection. *BMC Musculoskel Dis* 19:352
23. Lu J, Han J, Zhang C et al (2017) Infection after total knee arthroplasty and its gold standard surgical treatment: spacers used in two-stage revision arthroplasty. *Intractable Rare Dis Res* 6(4):256–261
24. Estrella EP, Eufemio EMT (2008) Isolated extensor hallucis longus paralysis after knee arthroscopy: a case report. *Foot Ankle J* 1(10):2
25. Yacub JN, Rice JB, Dillingham TR (2009) Nerve injury in patients following hip and knee arthroplasties and knee arthroscopy. *Am J Phys Med Rehabil* 88(8):635–691

Safe Leg Surgery

12

12.1 Introduction

Tibial fractures constitute a large number of emergency surgeries in most trauma centers. In fact, fractures of the tibial shaft are the most common injury treated by orthopaedic surgeons. Tibial shaft fractures account for 15% of all adult fractures and are often high-energy injuries. About 25% are open fractures with noteworthy soft tissue injury, which can be devastating. Moreover, these fractures are prone to complications. The tibia carries nearly five times body weight in axial force during walking. It is also plays an important role with bending and twisting forces, especially when the foot is placed on the ground, although its resistance against these loads is far less than with compression. The fibula accounts for 6–17% of the weight bearing load of the leg [1–6].

Most tibial shaft fractures in younger patients result from direct, high-energy mechanisms of injury. These injuries often cause a displaced, comminuted fracture that is frequently accompanied by considerable soft tissue damage. The anterior tibial artery is often damaged in tibia fractures and is the source of significant bleeding and elevated compartment pressure [7, 8].

The lack of a circumferential soft tissue envelope around the tibia contributes to challenges like infection and nonunion. Advanced bone reconstruction and soft tissue surgery is typically required to attain bone and soft tissue healing. As demonstrated well in the literature, the tibial nail is the most advantageous method, since it runs in the biomechanical axis of the lower limb and is minimally invasive. Although it was once used mainly for the tibial shaft fractures, recent advances in instrumentation and surgical technique have allowed this system to be used to treat fractures of the proximal and distal tibia also [9, 10]. Intramedullary nails have become the management of choice both for unstable closed fractures and for low-energy–induced fractures [11]. Success in correctly positioning the tibial nail depends on the location and on the insertion angle [11].

S. V. Babu, *Safe Orthopaedic Surgery*,
https://doi.org/10.1007/978-981-16-2846-7_12

Open tibial shaft fracture, caused by the strong direct force, is one of the most common fractures in road traffic accidents [12]. The rate of complications, including osteomyelitis, is much lower in patients who have complete soft tissue reconstruction performed within 72 h of open leg injuries [9]. External fixation is advocated for severe open fractures or in unstable polytraumatized patients for whom prolonged surgery could be harmful in damage-control orthopaedics [9, 12–17].

Proximal tibial fractures are caused by two mechanisms—either by strong impact, such as road accidents in young individuals, or by a relatively weak impact, such as a fall in elderly people. High-energy tibial plateau fractures are brutal injuries often associated with higher incidences of infection and soft tissue damages. Less invasive stabilization system (LISS) has become accepted for these fractures and offers apparent biomechanical advantages over traditional plating. LISS causes considerably less iatrogenic tissue damage, reduces perioperative complications, has a shorter operative time, and a lower rate of infection [18].

Distal tibia fractures are multifaceted injuries with an elevated complication rate. Many treatment modalities are available for these fractures, such as conventional open reduction and internal fixation, external fixation with or without limited internal fixation, intramedullary nailing, and minimally invasive plate osteosynthesis. All of these surgeries have their own advantages and disadvantages. Regardless, the goals of surgical management of leg fractures are to attain soft tissue healing, ensure a high-quality osseous union, reinstate the length of the limb and the proper arrangement of both bones and their particular joints, and achieve full range of pain-free function of the lower limb.

Tibial shaft fractures are the third most common long bone fractures in the pediatric age group, with an incidence of 15%. They are the second most common fractures requiring hospitalization, after femur fractures. The standard treatment of tibial shaft fractures in children is manipulation and casting. Surgical treatment is indicated for these fractures in polytrauma, neurovascular injury, and open injury, as well as in failure to obtain a satisfactory closed reduction. It is also beneficial in the stabilization of closed fracture after fasciotomy for compartment syndrome [19, 20].

While there is little literature on the incidence of isolated fibula shaft fractures, they typically occur as a result of direct injury in sports, road accident, or gunshot wound. They may be associated with superficial peroneal nerve injury, vascular injury, and compartment syndrome [21]. Children less than 8 years of age can tolerate 100% translation of the tibial shaft and up to 10° of sagittal and coronal angulation. However, there are surgical indications for these fractures [6, 22]. As established, the primary goal of surgical fixation of both bones of the leg, either by internal or external modalities, is to preserve the length and alignment and ensure no rotation of the fracture.

Nonoperative treatment may be advised for closed tibial shaft fractures when there is minimal soft tissue injury and when there is no substantial displacement or deformity of fracture. The upper limits of acceptable deformity are 5° of angulation in the coronal plane, 10° of angulation in the sagittal plane, 5° of rotational deformity, and less than 1 cm of shortening [2].

12.2 Applied Surgical Anatomy of the Leg

The leg has a multifarious anatomy comprising the tibia, the fibula, and their intraosseous membrane. They are well surrounded by important muscles within four compartments (anterior, lateral, superficial posterior, deep posterior) and by intimate neurovascular structures.

The tibia has a major subcutaneous region, making it easy to access. The fibula is much closer to the common peroneal nerve and its branches.

The deep fascia of the leg is a hard, fibrous, obstinate structure that encloses the calf muscle. Two intermuscular septa, one anterior and one posterior, pass from the deep surface of the encircling fascia to the fibula and fully envelope the peroneal compartment of the leg.

12.2.1 Common Peroneal Nerve

The common peroneal nerve begins posteriorly in the thigh and runs from the center of the popliteal fossa laterally and anteriorly together and below the tendon of the biceps femoris. It runs anteriorly around the neck of the fibula and then divides in the anterior compartment into superficial sensory, deep motor, and sensory branches.

12.2.2 Saphenous Nerve

The saphenous nerve is purely sensory. It runs distally on the anteromedial side of the thigh and passes the knee joint on the medial side of the patella, where it gives off the infrapatellar branch. At the ankle it is anterior to the medial malleolus, where it runs together with the long saphenous vein.

12.2.3 Popliteal Artery

The popliteal artery traverses the center of the popliteal fossa. It trifurcates at the level of the proximal tibial shaft into the anterior tibial artery, peroneal artery, and posterior tibial artery.

12.2.4 Knee Joint Capsule

Pin placement must respect the knee joint capsule and be placed 2 cm inferior to the tibial plateau. If more proximal pin fixation is needed for a very high fractures, it must be as anterior as possible because of the shorter extent of the knee joint capsule in this area.

12.2.5 Tibiofibular Joint

The common peroneal nerve runs around the fibular neck and then goes anteriorly and distally.

12.2.6 Distal to the Tibial Tuberosity

To reduce the risk of infection, it is best to insert the pins where soft tissue coverage is less. Therefore, distal to the tibial tubercle,- the safe zones for pin insertion are the tibial crest and the medial surface of the tibia. The surgeon has to be cautious and avoid deep penetration beyond the distal cortex.

The neurovascular bundle (the anterior tibial artery and vein together with the deep peroneal nerve) runs in front of the interosseous membrane close to the posterolateral border of the tibia. They are in danger if the pin is inserted in the direction about halfway between the anterior crest and the medial surface of the tibia.

12.3 Principles of Safe Tibia and Fibula Surgery [3, 11, 13, 23–30]

12.3.1 Safety Principles for the Anterolateral Approach to the Lateral Tibial Plateau

- The superficial branch of the peroneal nerve has an unpredictable course. Hence, utmost care is to be given while dissecting posteriorly in this region.
- The lateral meniscus is at most risk during incision of the synovium of the knee joint. It has to be carefully detached for adequate visualization of the articular surface of the tibia.

12.3.2 Safety Principles for Minimally Invasive Anterolateral Approach to the Proximal Tibia

- The superficial branch of the peroneal nerve, as mentioned, has a changeable course. To avoid injuring this nerve, care has to be given while dissecting in the posterior region.
- Excessive internal rotation of the insertion guide in the LISS must be avoided as it might endanger the popliteal artery.

12.3.3 Safety Principles for the Posteromedial Approach to the Proximal Tibia

- The saphenous nerve and vein pass through the superficial surgical dissection field and should be safeguarded.

12.3.4 Safety Principles for the Anterior Approach to the Tibia

- The long saphenous vein, which runs on the medial side of the calf, is vulnerable during superficial surgical dissection and must be preserved.

12.3.5 Safety Principles for Minimally Invasive Surgery of the Distal Tibia

- The periosteum covering the tibia is significant for the vascular supply of the bone. The plane that is between the periosteum and the subcutaneous tissues is used in this approach.

12.3.6 Safety Principles for the Posterolateral Approach to the Tibia

- The short saphenous vein may be injured when the skin flaps are mobilized.
- The branches of the peroneal artery cross the space between the gastrocnemius and peroneus brevis muscles.
- The posterior tibial artery and tibial nerve are well protected when the surgical dissection is on the interosseous membrane, and the surgeon should not go to the platform posterior to the flexor hallucis longus and tibialis posterior muscles.

12.3.7 Safety Principles for the Approach to the Fibula

- The common peroneal nerve is exposed as it goes around the neck of the fibula. The key to preserving the nerve is to visualize it proximally as it presents on the posterior border of the biceps femoris. It then can be safely traced through the peroneal belly. Retracting the nerve is to be avoided.
- The dorsal cutaneous branch of the superficial peroneal nerve is vulnerable to injury at the junction of the distal and middle thirds of the fibula.
- Subperiosteal dissection in the lateral malleolus region will prevent injury to the branches of the peroneal artery and the short saphenous vein.

12.3.8 Safety Principles for the Minimally Invasive Approach for Tibial Intramedullary Nailing

- The infrapatellar branch of the saphenous nerve is commonly damaged in this procedure.
- If a fracture table is used, the thigh rest is placed within the popliteal fossa. Compression of the popliteal vein can result and increase the risk of deep venous thrombosis.

- The incision can be lateral, medial parapatellar, or transpatellar in approaching the point of entry in the proximal tibia, but transpatellar is most common.
- Under imaging guidance, the ideal entry point is medial to the tibial spine in anteroposterior view and just adjacent to the anterior margin of the joint surface in the lateral view.
- In the frontal plane, the nail entry is present in line with the medullary canal (3 mm medial of the tibial crest). In the sagittal plane, the nail entry is located just distal to the angle between tibial plateau and anterior tibial metaphysis.
- If the entry of the tibial nail is too posterior, injury to the insertion of the anterior cruciate ligament on the tibia will result. An entry point that is too far anterior can cause splintering of the anterior cortex of the tibia during nail insertion.
- For intramedullary flexible nailing insertion in children, paramount care is be taken in avoiding physis injury. The entry point should be 2 cm away from the metaphysis.
- The titanium elastic nail system works by balancing the forces among the two opposite flexible implants. To attain this balance, the nail diameter must be 40% of the narrowest canal diameter (Flynn's equation: nail diameter = 0.4 × the diameter of the medullary canal), and the nails must assume a double C construct. Also, the nails must have a similar smooth curve with same level entry points. The nail end should be left proud and has to be less than 2 cm.

12.3.9 Safety Principles for Externally Fixation of the Tibia

- In pediatric tibial external fixation, the pins have to be placed 2 cm from the physis.
- In adults, any pin placed near a joint must be a minimum of 14 mm away from the joint line to prevent joint sepsis.
- For bridging external fixators, the pins are placed anteriorly in the tibial shafts.
- The anterior tibial artery and vein, along with the deep peroneal nerve, jointly travel anterior to the interosseous membrane much closer to the posterolateral border of the tibia.
- Pins must be inserted sufficiently deep to engage in the distal cortex. In the far cortex, the pins must not protrude, so as not to damage the neurovascular bundle or the soft tissues.
- Drilling a hole in the thick tibial crest will produce excessive heat, and there is danger that the drill bit can go any in direction, damaging the soft tissues. Since the anteromedial tibial surface provides sufficient thickness for the placement of pins, this approach is advised: The tibia is divided into three segments as illustrated (Fig. 12.1). An angle (relative to the sagittal plane) of 20–60° for the proximal fragment and of 30–90° for the distal fragment is suggested. Segment 1 should have the screws placed obliquely to avoid posterior tibial neurovascular bundle injury, segment 2 should have sagittal plane screwss and segment 3 screws must be anteroposterior at the plane between the lateral edge of the tibialis posterior and extensor hallucis longus.

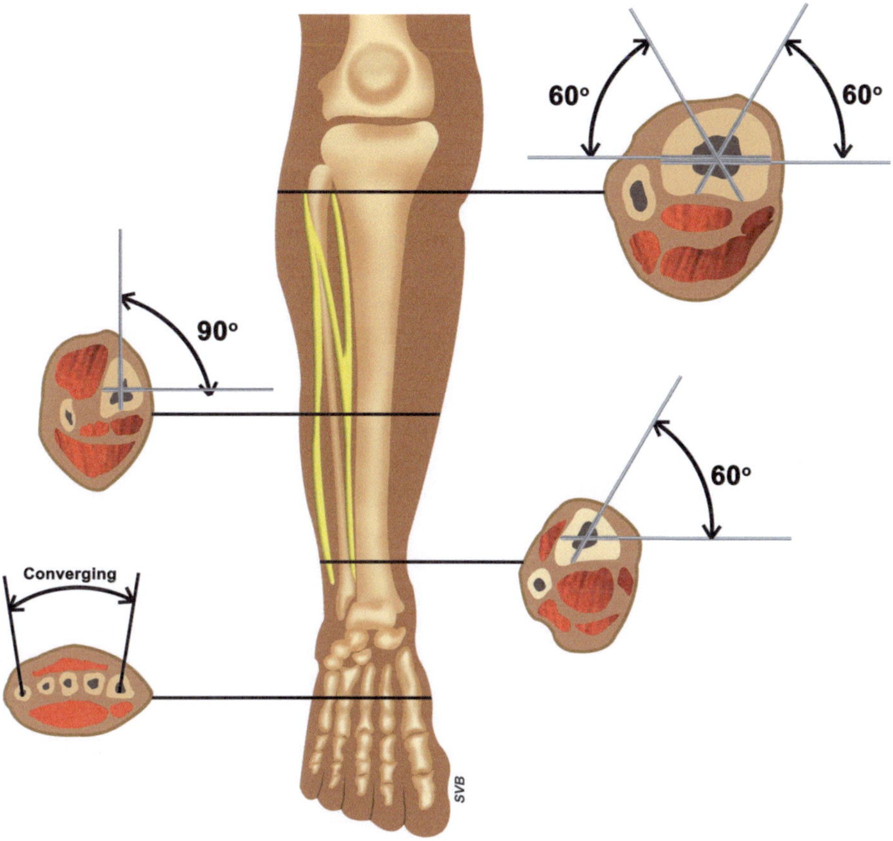

Fig. 12.1 The leg and its safe zones for external fixation

12.3.10 Safety Principles for Approaching the Compartments of the Leg

- To decompress the anterior and lateral compartments of the leg, a longitudinal incision is made on the anterolateral aspect of the lower leg. It should start at the level of tibial tubercle and extend up to 6 cm above the ankle. The fascia over the anterior and lateral compartments is incised in the line of skin incision.
- To decompress the superficial and deep posterior (flexor) compartments, a longitudinal incision is made on the posteromedial aspect of the lower leg. It starts at the point of the tibial tubercle and distally extends up to 6 cm above the ankle. Decompressing the deep posterior compartment involves lifting the soleus muscle from the intermuscular septum and dissecting the compartment under direct vision to prevent injury of the posterior neurovascular bundle

12.4 Discussion

Surgical complications have been reported in more than 30% of distal tibia fractures due to the marginal soft tissue and vascular supply in this area [31]. Plate fixation in distal metaphyseal fractures has more risk of delayed union or nonunion. However, a German study confirmed that surgical management with plate fixation had a complication rate of 12% compared with 25% for intramedullary nailing [26]. The complications of intramedullary nailing for distal-third tibial shaft and metaphyseal fractures have a direct effect on ankle and foot function. However, these can be well reduced by impacting the unreamed nail into the subchondral bone while maintaining the fracture reduction and also by using multiple distal locking screws in different planes [26]. Comorbid factors such as diabetes and peripheral arterial dysfunction can lead to significant complications [32].

The incidence of neurologic complications has been reported as high as 30% in reamed intramedullary nailing of the tibia [7]. Knee pain after nailing is a noted complication [33]. The incidence of iatrogenic damage to the infrapatellar nerve after tibial nailing is higher and long-lasting; injury to this nerve is always associated with anterior knee pain [33]. The incidence of septic complications after nailing of the tibia exceeds 6% [34]. Fracture healing is delayed in when there is vascular injury, and such injuries have to be managed well [35–37]. The oblique proximal locking screw used in tibial fracture nailing has produced peroneal nerve damage and significant morbidity after surgery [36]. Malrotation remains a generally documented complication after tibial nailing [3].

Because of the lack of soft tissue covering the tibia and its mechanical disadvantages, internal fixation with plates should be avoided if possible and be used only for tibial shaft nonunions or for fractures with articular or periarticular extension. External fixation can be used instead of intramedullary nailing in patients with severe soft tissue injury or in damage-control surgery in patients with polytrauma. If converting to an intramedullary nail, the procedure should be carried out at as early as possible, preferably within 4 weeks, to minimize the chance of pin sepsis [2].

LISS may be technically challenging, has a long learning curve, is expensive, and incurs higher radiation exposure. A new system, the U-grooved locking compression plate, has been used for proximal tibial fractures with a shorter operating time, less radiation exposure, lower cost, and good functional recovery than with LISS [30].

A Chinese study showed that external fixation is more effective than internal fixation in reducing hospitalization time and fracture healing time and in lowering the total complication rates of pediatric tibial shaft fractures [9]. Safe corridors and zones have been suggested to prevent neurovascular complications in external fixation surgery [16] (see Fig. 12.1). A safe zone refers to placement of thin wires so as to avoid neurovascular structures and intrasynovial placement to diminish the prospect of septic arthritis [14]. Any pin placed near a joint should be a minimum of 14 mm away from the joint line to prevent joint sepsis. The neurovascular structures around the knee (common peroneal nerve, deep peroneal nerve, and popliteal artery) must be avoided.

Although external fixation is advised in open pediatric tibial fractures, intramedullary flexible nailing can be safely performed with very low risk of wound or infectious challenges [38, 39]. The risk of compartment syndrome is higher, however, regardless of whether a child has a closed or open tibia fracture, and utmost care must be taken in performing flexible nailing in patients who may have associated closed head injury, due to a risk of systemic complications [40].

A combination of pins and flexible intramedullary nails is effectual in producing more stability and is not associated with more complications [41]. It is important that both flexible nails are of equal diameter, since differences will produce differential loading of opposite cortices and may lead to angular deformity. By principle, two flexible nails with three-point fixation are a simple load-sharing devices that will preserve alignment and rotation, will permit mobilization in producing bridging callus, and will not cross the physis. It is also straightforward to introduce and remove the nails after bony union. These benefits, plus shorter hospitalization, fewer complications, and excellent functional outcome, have led many surgeons to use this system to treat pediatric long bone fractures [19, 42].

Pin tract infection is a frequently expected problem, possibly even an unavoidable complication, when using external fixation, with very high incidence [14]. Biofilm-related bacterial infections are challenging, and *Staphylococcus aureus* is the most common organism. When applying the pins, they must not drilled on the soft tissues; they should be pushed into the near cortex, then drilled through the bone, and finally advanced through the opposite soft tissue by tapping with a mallet. Standardized pin site protocols that encompass a knowledge of external fixator biomechanics and detailed surgical technique during pin and wire insertion, postoperative pin site dressings, and pin removal could reduce the incidence of major infections and treatment malfunctions [43]. Secondary nailing after external fixation for tibial shaft fractures should be early, before onset of pin tract infection [44].

The incidence of vascular injury in open tibial fractures is 29%, and CT angiography is a useful tool in diagnosing vascular injuries that may require intervention [45]. Open fractures of the leg must be given utmost care by the orthoplastic systems, and proper documentation, including photography before debridement and at all key stages of management, is recommended [25, 46].

A comprehensive neurovascular examination must be performed and documented in all leg injuries [3]. Also, it is imperative to institute suitable interpersonal communications to ensure proper diagnosis and rule out other injuries that could influence a different, possibly surgical, treatment. This communication among surgeons, those in orthopaedics, and those in other specialties, can enhance patient-centered care and ultimately lead to improved outcomes.

The rate of infection and soft tissue breakdown is very high for both tibial shaft fractures and tibial plateau fractures, especially in for high-energy injuries. Utilizing small wires and hybrid external fixation has been reported to be more beneficial than plate osteosynthesis in these high-energy fractures [18].

Infection after tibial shaft fracture surgery is associated increased healthcare resource use and costs. The incidences of infection and nonunion have been significantly reduced with new treatment modalities, but these complications continue to be a source of considerable morbidity and mortality. While there are reports from some parts of the world of a 35% infection rate after tibial fracture surgery, a large multicenter recent study in India reported only a 3% rate of infection after internal fixation of open and closed tibia fractures. This study confirmed another Indian study that showed that the duration of prophylactic antibiotic usage is longer than accepted practice in other part of the world, raising concern for the possible development of antibiotic-resistant microbes within Indian orthopaedic settings. Antibiotic management should not exceed 72 h unless there is spreading sepsis [23, 46–53].

Advances in managing implant-related infections in tibial surgery include more developed external fixators, vancomycin cement, vacuum-assisted dressings, and use of perforator and other flaps in reconstructing the soft tissues. The amalgamation of these practices seems to produce promising results [54]. Moreover, it is highly recommended that all health establishments implement an antibiotic stewardship program and safety protocols to prevent and manage surgical site infections [47–49] (see also Chap. 1).

References

1. Madadi F, Eajazi A, Madadi F et al (2011) Adult tibial shaft fractures: different patterns, various treatments and complications. *Med Sci Monit* 17(11):CR640–CR645
2. Courtney PM, Berstein J, Ahn J (2011) In brief: closed tibial shaft fractures. *Clin Orthop Relat Res* 469(12):3518–3521
3. Zelle BA, Boni G (2015) Safe surgical technique: intramedullary nail fixation of tibial shaft fractures. *Patient Saf Surg* 9:40
4. Pahlevanhosseini H, Shahbazi-Bilehsavar F, Abrisham SM-J, Shafiee M (2017) Open tibial shaft fracture treatment with plating within 6 hours and between 6-24 hours after injury. *Bali Med J* 6(2):445–448
5. Doshi P, Gopalan H, Sprague S et al (2017) Incidence of infection following internal fixation of open and closed tibia fractures in India (INFINITI): a multi-centre observational cohort study. *BMC Musculoskel Dis* 18(1):156
6. Patel NK, Horstman J, Kuester V et al (2018) Pediatric tibial shaft fractures. *Indian J Orthop* 52(5):522–528
7. Koval KJ, Clapper MF, Brumback RJ et al (1991) Complications of reamed intramedullary nailing of the tibia. *J Orthop Trauma* 5(2):184–189
8. Erin-Madsen N, Aasvang TK, Viberg B et al (2019) Knee pain and associated complications after intramedullary nailing of tibial shaft fracture. *Dan Med J* 66(8):A5554
9. Lua JYC, Tan VH, Sivasubramanian H, Kwek EBK (2017) Complications of open fracture management: risk factors and treatment. *Malays Orthop J* 11(1):18–22
10. Pobłocki K, Domaradzki M (2011) Gawdzik, et al. Complications after intramedullary nailing of the tibia [article in Polish]. *Chir Narzadow Ruchu Ortop Pol* 76(5):274–277
11. Labronici PJ, Moreira IL Jr, Lyra FS, Franco JS (2010) Localization of the tibial entry point. *Rev Bras Ortop* 45(4):375–381
12. Golubović Z, Stojiljković P, Macukanović-Golubović L et al (2008) External fixation in the treatment of open tibial shaft fractures [article in Serbian]. *Vojnosanit Pregl* 65(5):343–348
13. Nayagam S (2007) Safe corridors in external fixation: the lower leg (tibia, fibula, hindfoot and forefoot). *Strat Trauma Limb Reconstr* 2(2-3):105–110
14. Schalamon J, Petnehazy T, Ainoedhofer H et al (2007) Pin tract infection with external fixation of pediatric fractures. *J Pediatr Surg* 42(9):1584–1587

15. Russo A-P, Caubere A, Ghabi A et al (2018) Sequential management of tibial fractures using a temporary unicortical external fixator. *SICOT J* 4:39
16. Qiu S, Liu J, Liu C (2017) Effects of external fixation technique on hospitalization time, fracture healing time and complication rate of pediatric fracture. *Int J Clin Exp Med* 10(8):12179–12185
17. Dar RA, Lal T, Maajid S et al (2019) Retrospective analysis on use of external fixation in pediatric extremity trauma and fractures as a damage control device and their outcome in a tertiary care set up. *Int J Orthop Sci* 5(1):292–294
18. Stannard JP, Finkemeier CG, Lee J, Kregor PJ (2008) Utilization of the less-invasive stabilization system internal fixator for open fractures of the proximal tibia: a multi-center evaluation. *Indian J Orthop* 42(4):426–430
19. Zarad AL (2014) Flexible intramedullary nails for unstable fractures of the tibia in children: a retrospective evaluation of effectiveness. *Egypt Orthop J* 49(4):281–285
20. Uludag A, Tosun HB (2019) Treatment of unstable pediatric tibial shaft fractures with titanium elastic nails. *Medicina (Kaunas)* 55(6):266
21. Walters BB, Constant D, Anand P (2021) Fibula fractures. *StatPearls [Internet]*. StatPearls Publishing, Treasure Island, FL
22. Srivastava AK, Mehlman CT, Wall EJ, Do TT (2008) Elastic stable intramedullary nailing of tibial shaft fractures in children. *J Pediatr Orthop* 28(2):152–158
23. World Health Organization. WHO guidelines for safe surgery: safe surgery saves lives. Published 2009. https://www.who.int/teams/integrated-health-services/patient-safety/research/safe-surgery&publication=9789241598552
24. Hoppenfeld S, de Boer P, Buckley R (2022) *Surgical exposures in orthopaedics: the anatomic approach*, 6th edn. Wolters Kluwer, Philadelphia
25. Nanchahal J, Nayagam S, Khan U et al (2009) Standards for the management of open fractures of the lower limb. British Association of Plastic, Reconstructive and Aesthetic Surgeons (BAPRAS). https://www.bapras.org.uk/docs/default-source/commissioning-and-policy/standards-for-lower-limb.pdf?sfvrsn=0
26. Yaligod V, Rudrappa GH, Nagendra S, Shivanna UM (2014) Minimizing the complications of intramedullary nailing for distal third tibial shaft and metaphyseal fractures. *J Orthop* 11(1):10–18
27. Humphrey JA, Gillani S, Barry MJ (2015) The role of external fixators in paediatric trauma. *Acta Orthop Belg* 81(3):363–367
28. British Orthopaedic Association (BOA), British Association of Plastic, Reconstructive and Aesthetic Surgeons (BAPRAS). Audit standards for trauma: open fractures. Published 2017. https://www.boa.ac.uk/uploads/assets/3b91ad0a-9081-4253-92f7d90e8df0fb2c/29bf80f1-1cb6-46b7-afc761119341447f/open%20fractures.pdf
29. AO Surgery Reference. Published 2019. https://www2.aofoundation.org/wps/portal/surgery
30. Yin B, Chen W, Zhang Q et al (2012) Tibial fracture treated by minimally invasive plating using a novel low-cost, high-technique system. *Int Orthop* 36(8):1687–1693
31. Joveniaux P, Ohl X, Harisboure A et al (2010) Distal tibia fractures: management and complications of 101 cases. *Int Orthop* 34(4):583–588
32. Neumann MV, Strohm PC, Reising K et al (2016) Complications after surgical management of distal lower leg fractures. *Scand J Trauma Resusc Emerg Med* 24:146
33. Leliveld MS, Verhofstad MHJ (2012) Injury to the infrapatellar branch of the saphenous nerve, a possible cause for anterior knee pain after tibial nailing? *Injury* 43(6):779–783
34. Greibauer M, Kaltenecker G, Vécsei V (1995) Septic complications after interlocking nailing of the tibia. *Eur J Orthop Surg Traumatol* 5(1):65–68
35. Brinker MR, Bailey DE Jr (1997) Fracture healing in tibia fractures with an associated vascular injury. *J Trauma* 42(1):11–19
36. Brinker MR, Caines MA, Kerstein MD, Elliott MN (2000) Tibial shaft fractures with an associated infrapopliteal arterial injury: a survey of vascular surgeons opinions on the need for vascular repair. *J Orthop Trauma* 14(3):194–198

37. Drosos GI, Stavropoulos NI, Kazakos KI (2007) Peroneal nerve damage by oblique proximal locking screw in tibial fracture nailing: a new emerging complication? *Arch Orthop Trauma Surg* 127(6):449–451
38. Ahmed KFE, Zakaria B, Hadhood M, Shaheen A (2014) Management of diaphyseal tibial fracture in pediatrics by elastic stable intramedullary nails. *Menoufia Med J* 27(2):401–406
39. Heo J, Oh C-W, Park K-H et al (2016) Elastic nailing of tibia shaft fractures in young children up to 10 years of age. *Injury* 47(4):832–836
40. Pandya NK, Edmonds EW (2012) Immediate intramedullary flexible nailing of open pediatric tibial shaft fractures. *J Pediatr Orthop* 32(8):770–776
41. Aslani H, Tabrizi A, Sadighi A, Mirblok AR (2013) Treatment of open pediatric tibial fractures by external fixation versus flexible intramedullary nailing: a comparative study. *Arch Trauma Res* 2(3):108–112
42. Patil C, J A (2019) Study of the outcome of titanium elastic nail system (TENS) in diaphyseal fractures of femur and tibia in children. *Int J Orthop Sci* 5(3):617–620
43. Roussignol X, Sigonney G, Potage D et al (2015) Secondary nailing after external fixation for tibial shaft fracture: risk factors for union and infection: a 55 case series. *Orthop Traumatol Surg Res* 101(1):89–92
44. Ceroni D, Grumetz C, Desvachez O et al (2016) From prevention of pin-tract infection to treatment of osteomyelitis during paediatric external fixation. *J Child Orthop* 10:605–612
45. O'Malley O, Trompeter AJ, Krishnanandan S et al (2019) How common are vascular injuries in open tibial fractures? A prospective longitudinal cohort study. *Eur J Orthop Surg Traumatol* 29(5):1119–1124
46. National Institute for Health and Care Excellence. Open fractures in hospital. NICE Pathways, 2021. https://pathways.nice.org.uk/pathways/trauma/open-fractures-in-hospital
47. National Institute for Health and Care Excellence. Antimicrobial stewardship: systems and processes for effective antimicrobial medicine use. NICE guideline 15. Published August 18, 2015. https://www.nice.org.uk/guidance/ng15
48. Seligman KM, Katz D, Farber MK (2018) Preventing surgical site infection after cesarean delivery: the anesthesia professional's role. *APSF Newsletter* 33(1):25–27
49. National Institute for Health and Care Excellence. Surgical site infections: prevention and treatment. NICE guideline 125. Published 2020. https://www.nice.org.uk/guidance/ng125
50. World Health Organization. Antimicrobial stewardship programmes in health-care facilities in low- and middle-income countries: a WHO practical toolkit. Published 2019. https://apps.who.int/iris/handle/10665/329404
51. Whiting PS, Galat DD, Zirkle LG et al (2019) Risk factors for infection after intramedullary nailing of open tibial shaft fractures in low- and middle-income countries. *J Orthop Trauma* 33(6):e234–e239
52. Chitnis AS, Canderkarr M, Sparks C et al (2019) Complications and its impact in patients with closed and open tibial shaft fractures requiring open reduction and internal fixation. *J Comp Eff Res* 8(16):1405–1416
53. Farooqui HH, Mehta A, Selvaraj S (2019) Outpatient antibiotic prescription rate and pattern in the private sector in India: evidence from medical audit data. *PLoS One* 14(11):e0224848
54. Xu Y-Q, Zhu Y-L, Fan X-Y et al (2014) Implant-related infection in the tibia: surgical revision strategy with vancomycin cement. *Sci World J* 2014:124864

13 Safe Ankle and Foot Surgery

13.1 Introduction

The goal of ankle surgery is to provide pain relief and functional improvement. Any slight imperfection in the ankle will create much alteration in both gait and biomechanics of the foot and ankle.

Surgical treatment for ankle fracture is a common orthopaedic procedure. Ankle fracture incidence had risen appreciably in the last decades, most commonly affecting two age groups: high-energy injury in young patients and low-energy insult in elderly patients. Open reduction and internal fixation (ORIF) represents the gold standard in the management of ankle fractures for reinstating anatomic alignment and articular congruity of the ankle mortise for avoiding altered loading to the tibiotalar joint and the consequent poor functional results. Although results are generally favorable, postoperative complications are not unusual (incidence of 1–40%) and have a substantial impact on postoperative morbidity, worsening of the quality of life and increasing healthcare costs. The most litigations for these complications have occurred in the United Kingdom [1–3].

Approaches to the structures of the ankle and foot typically are straightforward; the bones and joints that are explored normally are superficial. Apart from technical struggles associated with the surgery itself, the most common complication in foot and ankle surgery is poor wound healing. For this reason, it is important to study both the circulation and the sensation of the foot well before surgery. Ischemic or neuropathic feet heal poorly and are a common contraindication to elective surgery. Elderly and diabetic patients are at a higher risk of complications. In patients with comorbid factors like diabetes, ischemia and neuropathy must be evaluated carefully before any foot surgery is performed. Smoking is also a relative contraindication to surgery, especially in cases of ORIF for fractures of the calcaneus.

Wound healing also is affected by the thickness of the skin flaps that are raised; it is important to make these flaps as thick possible. Forceful retraction is to be

S. V. Babu, *Safe Orthopaedic Surgery*,
https://doi.org/10.1007/978-981-16-2846-7_13

avoided. Longer incisions require less forceful retraction to achieve identical exposure, so they are safer than short incisions.

After residual ankle pain and posttraumatic ankle osteoarthritis, postoperative wound infection is the most common complication of ankle fracture surgery. The overall surgical site infection rate reported in the literature ranges from 1.4% to as high as 13% [2]. The surgeon should follow the guidelines from the World Health Organization and other International forums in preventing surgical site infections [4–6].

Arthroscopy of the foot and ankle region has proved to be an imperative diagnostic and therapeutic tool problems in the far lower extremities. As the indications for arthroscopy have increased, complications associated with foot and ankle arthroscopy have also increased [7].

Total ankle arthroplasty offers a practical alternative to ankle arthrodesis in carefully selected patients. It has a steep learning curve but can yield good results when performed by a surgeon with good experience and training [8].

13.2 Applied Surgical Anatomy of the Foot and Ankle

The significant neurovascular structures in the forepart of the foot all are on the plantar side of the metatarsal bones, so they remain safeguarded (Fig. 13.1). The medial and lateral plantar arteries and nerves are present between the first and second layers of foot muscles. They are well protected by the overlying plantar fascia.

Dorsal incisions are preferred since they avoid cutting through the specialized weight-bearing region of the sole of the foot.

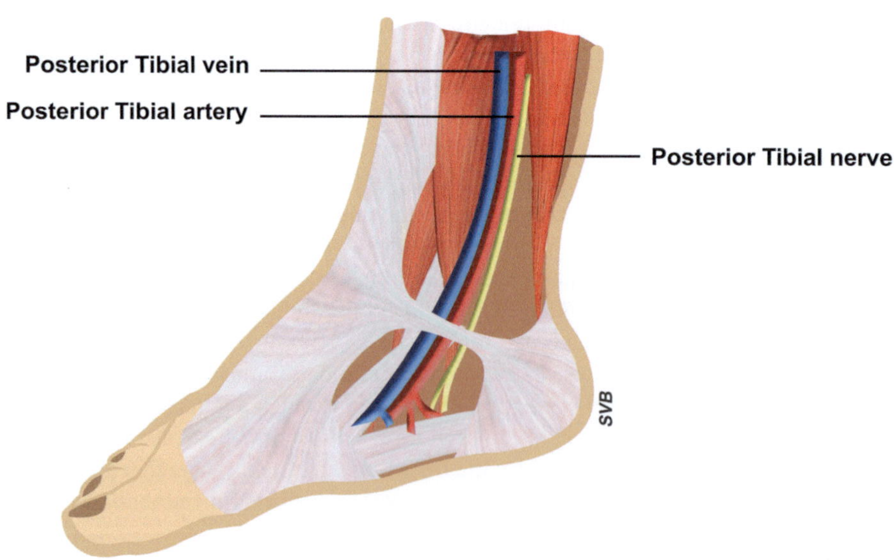

Fig. 13.1 The foot and its neurovascular relations

The abductor hallucis originates from the medial tubercle of the calcaneus and inserts into the medial side of the proximal phalanx of the great toe, and abducts the great toe. It is the only muscle that opposes the deformity of hallux valgus. The adductor hallucis, which attaches into the proximal phalanx via the lateral sesamoid bone, is the most important deforming force in hallux valgus. Many operations for this condition involve dissecting the muscle from its insertion and reinserting it into the head of the metatarsal so that it can act as a dynamic corrector of metatarsus varus.

13.3 Principles of Safe Foot and Ankle Surgery [9–15]

13.3.1 Safety Principles for the Anterior Approach to the Ankle

- The cutaneous branches of the superficial peroneal nerve travel close to the line of the ankle incision just under the skin. They must be protected during incision of the skin.
- The deep peroneal nerve and anterior tibial artery (the anterior neurovascular bundle) are to be noted and conserved during superficial surgical dissection. They are at great risk during skin incision, because they are very superficial and travel very close to the incision itself.
- Above the ankle joint, the neurovascular bundle is present between the tendons of the extensor hallucis longus and tibialis anterior muscles. At the level of the joint, the tendon of the extensor hallucis longus crosses over the bundle. The space between the tibialis anterior and the extensor hallucis longus can be used as long as the neurovascular bundle is recognized and mobilized to protect it.

13.3.2 Safety Principles for the Anterior and Posterior Approaches to the Medial Malleolus

- During the anterior incision, the saphenous nerve is in danger. It needs to be identified and preserved along with long saphenous vein.
- While making the posterior incision, care must be taken of many important structures that travel behind the medial malleolus—the tibialis posterior muscle, the flexor digitorum longus muscle, the posterior tibial artery and vein, the tibial nerve, and the flexor hallucis longus tendon.
- Leaving as much soft tissue attached to fractured malleolar fragments as possible is advised; complete dissection renders fragments avascular.

13.3.3 Safety Principles for the Medial Approach to the Ankle

- The saphenous nerve and the long saphenous vein are to be protected as a unit.

- The tendon of the tibialis posterior muscle is in danger during this approach, because it lies immediately below the medial malleolus.
- The tendons of the flexor hallucis longus and flexor digitorum longus muscle, together with the posterior neurovascular bundle, lie posterior and lateral to the medial malleolus.

13.3.4 Safety Principles for the Posteromedial Approach to the Ankle

- The posterior tibial artery and the tibial nerve (the posterior neurovascular bundle) are exposed during this approach. Forceful retraction is to be avoided.
- It should be borne in mind that the tibial nerve is unexpectedly large in young children and that the tendon of the flexor digitorum longus muscle is exceptionally small.

13.3.5 Safety Principles for the Posterolateral Approach to the Ankle

- The short saphenous vein and the sural nerve travel closely together. They should be protected as one unit.

13.3.6 Safety Principles for the Minimally Invasive Approach and Arthroscopic Ankle Surgery

- Minimally invasive technique is an alternative to the traditional method of ORIF. It allows for proper stabilization with minimal soft tissue traumatization, and thus could be recommended for patients with coexisting massive injuries affecting soft tissues and for those who do not agree to open reductions for cosmetic reasons. It allows for reduction of operative time and hospital stay. Nevertheless, it involves higher exposure to fluoroscopy and, in some cases, widening of the surgical approach.
- Surgeries have to be performed in hypoperfusion, after washing and typical dressing of surgical field. Following anatomic reduction under X-ray guidance, the lateral malleolus is stabilized with two or, in case of wide marrow cavity, three Kirschner wires. Then, after repositioning, the medial malleolus is fixed with one or two malleolar screws inserted laterally and posteriorly at a 30° angle through a 5-mm incision located over the superior aspect of the malleolus.
- If injured, the distal tibiofibular syndesmosis has to be reduced and stabilized under X-ray guidance with a single cortical screw with a 5-mm gasket through the access located superiorly to the syndesmosis. If necessary, the posterior mar-

gin of the tibia has to be reduced and fixed percutaneously under fluoroscopic guidance with a sharp single-tooth hook, stabilizing the bone fragment with a cortical screw or screws inserted through point incisions made on the anterolateral and anteromedial surfaces of the shin.

- There are three anterior and three posterior arthroscopic portals for ankle surgery. The anteromedial portal, the safest of all portals, is to be created first, just medial to the tendon of the anterior tibialis at or just proximal to the joint line. The anterolateral portal is created next, just lateral to the tendon of the peroneus tertius at or just proximal to the level of the joint line. An anterocentral portal can be made in the center of the ankle joint, but because of the major risks to the dorsalis pedis artery and vein and to the deep branch of the peroneal nerve, the use of this portal should be avoided if possible.
- The posterior portals are the posterolateral, trans-Achilles, and posteromedial portals. Of the posterior portals, the posterolateral portal is considered to be the safest, as there is less risk of damage to the Achilles tendon and to the posterior tibial nerve and vessels. The posterolateral portal is typically created by placing the arthroscope in the anteromedial portal inferior to the medial tibial notch and, under direct vision, using a long needle to make the portal entry just medial to the transverse tibiofibular ligament.
- The posteromedial portal is established with the help of the anterolateral and trans-Achilles portals in a straightforward approach. Finally, transmalleolar portals are made for Kirschner wire drilling of defects of the talar dome if needed.
- In general, the combination of the anteromedial, anterolateral, and posterolateral portals provides an excellent view of the entire joint. With the three-portal system, adequate inflow can be sustained by gravity drainage with use of lactated Ringer's solution; there is no need for an arthroscopic pump.

13.3.7 Safety Principles for the Lateral Approach to the Lateral Malleolus

- The sural nerve is susceptible when the skin flaps are mobilized in this approach. The terminal branches of the peroneal artery present immediately below the medial surface of the distal fibula.

13.3.8 Safety Principles for the Anterolateral Approach to the Ankle and Hind Part of the Foot

- The deep peroneal nerve and anterior tibial artery travel in front of the ankle joint. They are at risk if dissection is not carried out as close to the bone as possible.

13.3.9 Safety Principles for the Lateral Approach to the Hind Part of the Foot

- Exposures in this area are notorious for producing necrosis of skin flaps. Therefore, skin flaps are to be made as thick as possible, and dissection and retraction should be kept as thick as possible. Incisions should be kept as small as possible, and sharp curves are to be avoided.

13.3.10 Safety Principles for the Lateral Approach to the Posterior Talocalcaneal Joint

- The sural nerve is at risk in this approach. While mobilizing the skin, utmost care is needed to protect this nerve.

13.3.11 Safety Principles for the Lateral Approach to the Calcaneus

- The sural nerve is in danger if the skin flap is too proximally placed. The soft tissues are susceptible during this approach. The chance of skin necrosis can be minimized if the flap is dissected as a full-thickness flap since the skin derives its blood supply from the tissues underneath.
- Operations in this region may have to be delayed for a lengthy period to permit soft tissue swelling to reduce before surgery is undertaken.

13.3.12 Safety Principles for the Dorsal and Dorsomedial Approaches to the Metatarsophalangeal Joint of the Great Toe (Hallux Valgus Surgery)

- The tendon of the extensor hallucis longus muscle, which is present in the lateral edge of the wound, has to be acknowledged in this surgery. Indeed, in cases of bunion, the tendon bowstrings laterally over the metatarsophalangeal joint and becomes even more lateral to the incision than normal. The dorsal digital nerve is to be protected along the line of the incision.
- The tendon of the flexor hallucis longus muscle is exposed as the base of the proximal phalanx is dissected. The tendon presents in a groove on the plantar surface of the proximal phalanx much closer to the periosteum; if care is not taken, it can be damaged during dissection. The tendon is frequently displaced laterally in patients with hallux valgus.

13.3.13 Safety Principles for the Dorsal Approach to the Metatarsophalangeal Joints of the Second, Third, Fourth and Fifth Toes

- The long extensor tendon should be safeguarded during this surgery.
- At the level of the metatarsophalangeal joints, the plantar nerves and vessels are present in between the metatarsal heads, deep to the deep transverse metatarsal ligament. As long as the dissection is present over the dorsal aspect of the ligaments, the nerves are safe. Dissection around the metatarsal heads and proximal phalanges is to be carried out so as to prevent damage to the nerves and vessels that supply the weight-bearing area of the toes.

13.3.14 Safety Principles for the Approach to the Dorsal Web Spaces

- The only danger in this procedure is injury to the digital nerves and vessels. We need to take utmost care of these structures, which run under the incision. If more clefts must be explored, avoid disrupting the arterial supply to the toes. Accidental incision of one digital artery does not make a toe ischemic, but if the second digital artery to the same toe is injured in the adjacent web space, ischemia may result.

13.4 Discussion

Diagnostic arthroscopy of the ankle will be systematic and reproducible if the surgeon is well-informed about the intra-articular and extra-articular anatomy of the ankle and takes utmost care in placing the arthroscopic portals accurately and using a consistent technique. An eight-point arthroscopic surgery of the ankle has been suggested to make certain systematic and methodical evaluations of all areas of the ankle. The eight-point anterior examination is the study of the deltoid ligament; the medial gutter; the medial, central, and lateral aspects of the talus; the talofibular articulation; the lateral gutter; and the anterior gutter. The three-point central examination of arthroscopy covers the medial, central, and lateral portions of the tibiotalar joint. The seven-point posterior arthroscopy examines the medial gutter; the medial, central, and lateral aspects of the talus; the talofibular articulation; the lateral gutter; and the posterior gutter and lateral aspects of the talus; the talofibular articulation; the lateral gutter; and the posterior gutter . For the detailed and lengthier procedures, the surgeon must have the detailed anatomic knowledge of ankle and perfect skills for safe surgery [9, 11]. The evidence-based indications for ankle arthroscopy are management of ankle impingement, osteochondral lesions, and ankle arthrodesis. There is insufficient supported evidence for arthroscopy in managing ankle synovitis, fractures, or arthritis [16].

Open surgical fixation of ankle fracture affords a satisfying surgical treatment. However, complications are common, including posttraumatic arthritis and residual pain. Infection and impaired wound healing can be prevented if well addressed [16, 17]. It is highly recommended that all health establishments implement an antibiotic stewardship program and safety protocols to prevent and manage surgical site infections [4–6, 18, 19] (see also Chap. 1).

Ankle fusion has conventionally been the gold standard treatment for end-stage ankle arthritis. Improvements in prosthetic design and encouraging short- to medium-term results have increased interest in total ankle arthroplasty, however. The ideal patient for ankle arthroplasty is middle-aged or elderly and has an anatomically aligned ankle and heel, and their ankle has relatively preserved range of movement with at least 5° of dorsiflexion. Thus, ankle replacement is not a choice for every patient [8, 20].

References

1. Leyes M, Torres R, Guillén P (2003) Complications of open reduction and internal fixation of ankle fractures. *Foot Ankle Clin* 8(1):131–147
2. Mehta SS, Rees K, Cutler L, Mangwani J (2014) Understanding risks and complications in the management of ankle fractures. *Indian J Orthop* 48(5):445–452
3. Ovaska M (2015) Complications in ankle fracture surgery. *Acta Orthop Suppl* 86(358):1–32
4. World Health Organization. Antimicrobial stewardship programmes in health-care facilities in low- and middle-income countries: a WHO practical toolkit. Published 2019. https://apps.who.int/iris/handle/10665/329404
5. National Institute for Health and Care Excellence. Surgical site infections: prevention and treatment. NICE guideline 125. Published 2020. https://www.nice.org.uk/guidance/ng125
6. Seligman KM, Katz D, Farber MK (2018) Preventing surgical site infection after cesarean delivery: the anesthesia professional's role. *APSF Newsletter* 33(1):25–27
7. Deng DF, Hamilton GA, Lee M et al (2012) Complications associated with foot and ankle arthroscopy. *Foot Ankle Surg* 51(3):281–284
8. Syed F, Ugwuoke A (2018) Ankle arthroplasty: a review and summary of results from joint registries and recent studies. *EFORT Open Rev* 3(6):391–397
9. Andrews JR, Previte WJ, Carson WG (1985) Arthroscopy of the ankle: technique and normal anatomy. *Foot Ankle* 6(1):29–33
10. Gumann G (1987) Ankle arthroscopic portals and intra-articular anatomy. *J Foot Surg* 26(1):13–21
11. Gupta RK, Kansay RK, Aggarwal V et al (2008) Ankle arthroscopy: indications and techniques: a review article. *Pb J Orthop* X(1):66–71
12. van Dijk CN, van Bergen CJA (2008) Advancements in ankle arthroscopy. *J Am Acad Orthop Surg* 16(11):635–646
13. Hoppenfeld S, de Boer P, Buckley R (2022) Surgical exposures in orthopaedics: the anatomic approach, 6th edn. Wolters Kluwer, Philadelphia
14. Szczęsny G, Janowicz J (2012) Minimally invasive osteosynthesis of ankle fractures. *Pol Orthop Traumatol* 77:145–150
15. Gonzalez T, Chien B, Ghorbanhoseini M, Kwon JY (2017) Minimally invasive surgical approach to distal fibula fractures: a technique tip. *Arch Bone Jt Surg* 5(1):39–45
16. Glazebrook MA, Ganapathy V, Bridge MA et al (2009) Evidence-based indications for ankle arthroscopy. *Arthroscopy* 25(12):1478–1490

17. Macera A, Carulli C, Sirleo L, Innocenti M (2018) Postoperative complications and reoperation rates following open reduction and internal fixation of ankle fracture. *Joints* 6(2):110–115
18. National Institute for Health and Care Excellence. Antimicrobial stewardship: systems and processes for effective antimicrobial medicine use. NICE guideline 15. Published August 18, 2015. https://www.nice.org.uk/guidance/ng15
19. World Alliance for Patient Safety. Safe surgery saves lives: the second global safety challenge. World Health Organization website. Published 2009. https://www.who.int/patientsafety/safesurgery/knowledge_base/SSSL_Brochure_finalJun08.pdf
20. Bonasia DE, Dettoni F, Femino JE et al (2010) Total ankle replacement: why, when and how? *Iowa Orthop J* 30:119–130

MIX
Papier aus verantwortungsvollen Quellen
Paper from responsible sources
FSC® C105338

If you have any concerns about our products,
you can contact us on
ProductSafety@springernature.com

In case Publisher is established outside the EU,
the EU authorized representative is:
Springer Nature Customer Service Center GmbH
Europaplatz 3, 69115 Heidelberg, Germany

Printed by Libri Plureos GmbH
in Hamburg, Germany